There are numerous forms of depression. The science of the brain still has so many unknowns, yet many people can find a manageable solution within three to twelve months. Many will take longer, and some struggle to ever find a remedy. This is just my story. Everyone is different. But talking about it, confronting it, is the first step.

Andrew Robb

BLACK DOG DAZE

Public Life, Private Demons

Andrew Robb

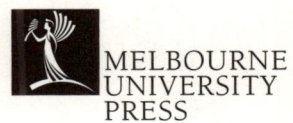

MELBOURNE
UNIVERSITY
PRESS

MELBOURNE UNIVERSITY PRESS
An imprint of Melbourne University Publishing Limited
187 Grattan Street, Carlton, Victoria 3053, Australia
mup-info@unimelb.edu.au
www.mup.com.au

First published 2011
Text © Andrew Robb, 2011
Design and typography © Melbourne University Publishing Limited, 2011

Cover design by Dave Altheim
Typeset by Megan Ellis
Printed by Griffin Press, South Australia

National Library of Australia Cataloguing-in-Publication entry
Robb, Andrew, 1951–
Black dog daze / Andrew Robb.

9780522858570 (pbk)
9780522860405 (ebook)

Includes index.

Liberal Party of Australia.
Politicians—Australia—Biography.
Depressed persons—Australia—Biography.

320.92

CONTENTS

INTRODUCTION

When you are sounded out to stand for leader of your political party, there can only be one answer.

I had been the Federal Director and Campaign Director for the Liberal Party for seven years from 1990. I had run John Hewson's campaign in 1993 and then John Howard's in 1996. Business commitments meant I wasn't free to consider preselection for a seat in the 2001 election, but happily I was elected to the federal seat of Goldstein in the 2004 election.

Although I had ambitions for a senior role, I needed time to learn about the parliamentary process, but time is what I didn't have. I needed to learn on the job, and fast.

I became chairman of the government's Workplace Relations Taskforce in 2005. The following years I was appointed Parliamentary Secretary with ministerial responsibilities for Immigration and Multicultural Affairs. I became the Minister for Vocational and Further Education in 2007, but then we lost the election. That wasn't part of the plan, but it was the risk I took.

I became Shadow Minister for Foreign Affairs, a wonderful portfolio, but not one I judged would be front and square in the 2010 election. In 2008 I became Shadow Minister for Infrastructure and Climate Change. These were significant positions but still down the food chain. And we were still in Opposition.

Then Godwin Grech torpedoed Malcolm Turnbull's leadership. The Treasury official had masqueraded as a reliable source for one or two people in the Liberal Party for two or three years, but then he forged an email that suggested Prime Minister Kevin Rudd and Treasurer Wayne Swan had acted improperly. Malcolm had seized on the apparent email to demand that the Prime Minister resign if he couldn't immediately justify his action.

Malcolm had desired the prime minister's job for much of his life. He felt well equipped to do it, and perhaps saw an opportunity for a single shot at bringing down the government, which also offered a more attractive alternative than the long, arduous political critique that is the job of the Opposition.

But Malcolm was duped and his credibility took an enormous hit. Politics is driven by symbols. For many, this became a powerful image of Malcolm's political judgement. Many Liberals thought that he did not have the qualities to be prime minister if he was going to take those sorts of risks. As a consequence, morale within the parliamentary party was at an all-time low.

In June 2009, the last week before we rose for the winter break, there was a lot of corridor talk and concern about Malcolm and the hit he and the party had taken. Everyone was examining tea leaves to see what the implications were: none of it looked positive. We had been browbeaten about Godwin at every opportunity in parliament that week.

Prime Minister Kevin Rudd was popular. He had studiously avoided offending anyone, as well as throwing literally tens of billions of dollars at the government's politically-inspired stimulus packages developed in response to the global financial crisis (GFC).

INTRODUCTION

The economy was showing signs of great resilience, and the feeling was that we could be in the political wilderness for a long time.

Parliament was rising on the Thursday. Everyone was talking. Everyone was trying to take the temperature. That afternoon I was talking to Victorian MP Tony Smith in the corridor about the situation. We agreed to meet again after 5 p.m. in my office. We quickly reached the conclusion that, according to the general consensus, things were terminal for Malcolm. I hadn't canvassed much among the Leadership group that week, but it certainly was the feeling of the majority of colleagues that if Malcolm stayed as leader, it would provide a very potent point of attack that would seriously undermine any chance of success at the next election. We were already a long way behind in the polls. We were also dealing with the highly divisive issue of the emissions trading scheme. Everyone was shell-shocked. There was likely to be an election within twelve to fifteen months. There was a lot of pessimism around and people were starting to ask: would we be more competitive with another leader?

The next move wasn't obvious. The best-known contenders were Tony Abbott and Joe Hockey. Joe would tell anyone who would listen that he didn't want it at this stage, and many thought Joe wasn't ready for higher office. Likewise, Tony himself felt he needed more time to broaden his appeal.

Tony Smith was direct: 'You'll have to consider it. Would you be interested?' There could be only one answer. I'd always felt that I could perform in leadership positions; that I had the skills, experience and character to do these jobs. Up until that point I had been a back-room player, but now I wanted to see how far I could go.

I had run national organisations for over twenty years and as federal director I did a lot of public work, but I needed to prove my capacity to carry a large body of people with me; to articulate a vision for the country and then convince Australians of its merit.

But I had come late to the parliament, aged fifty-three, and with five portfolios in six years, climate change was the only contentious area that placed me in the public domain arguing an alternative point of view. And even in that area, the battle was only just beginning, and I was moving in the opposite direction to our leader. Carrying an argument in a hostile political environment is a critical component of the top leadership, and whether I could hold my own in that area was untested.

Increasingly, I was engaged and acquitting myself more in the parliamentary and media debates. I was starting to believe that I could be effective in a public sense, so I wanted a leadership job. All I needed was to convince myself that I had the full armoury of necessary qualities.

Tony Smith was the first to ask, but then others posed the same question: would I consider mounting a challenge against Malcolm? There could be only one answer. I gave it then and I repeated it on a number of occasions in the following weeks: yes, I was interested, but I'd need to think about it.

I was very interested, but I had a problem.

1

THE PROBLEM

It had been a family joke, since our children were young, that I was 'not a morning person'. My wife, Maureen, would tell people that before 8.30 a.m. we didn't discuss the state of our marriage, and the kids wouldn't ask for money.

I had felt as if I had to make a transition from the leftovers of sleep into daily activity since I was a teenager. I needed to be quiet for a bit, to warm up to people, to get my head around ideas. I lacked confidence and felt very reluctant to make decisions. These needs weren't to be ignored and I had developed many strategies to manage them: long hot showers, sunshine, sneezing, the adrenaline rush of having to do a radio interview.

Typically this black mood would lift around 8 a.m. or 8.30 a.m. each morning, so it was irritating but manageable. But once I turned fifty I was aware this morning funk had become harder to shake. Nine o'clock, ten o'clock …

My staff, especially over the last twenty years, knew that I would be difficult to engage in the morning. They all knew not to interrupt me too early unless they really had too. Sometimes I got snappy, but most times it was just my body language saying, 'go away'. I would walk into the office and try to say hello to everybody in an effort to force myself out of it, but then I would retreat into my office and a lot of the times I closed the door.

I would try to schedule meetings after 9.30 a.m. Before then I would just be reading papers or briefs or doing something where I didn't have to talk to anybody. I could read, but I could never watch morning television. When I awoke each morning, I would listen to the 6 a.m. news and then turn the radio off. It annoyed me intensely: the voices, the noise, and I didn't want to be concerned with the trivial conversations of morning radio hosts.

Now I was responsible for the climate change policy. It was enormously interesting but it was a huge amount of work. I had to get on top of a mountain of detail. There were lots of meetings, speeches to give and press conferences. Some days I would have five, six, seven meetings, and four of them might be before midday, and yet I would be feeling flat and not in good form. It was *so* annoying. I'd be working really hard to engage properly, but it became more difficult and increasingly frustrating, and I suspect it detracted from my effectiveness.

This was the problem that stopped me jumping at the chance for the leadership. Although the little black dog that visited me every morning had been easily explained away as an aversion to mornings, after four decades I had finally admitted to myself earlier in the year that there might be more to it and consulted a GP, which turned out to be no help at all.

I explained the history and the symptoms and asked if there was a pill that might help. He just tapped his head and said it was all in my mind. Things just got comedic. He sent me to a local psychologist, who sat me on a couch in her front parlour. I started to recite the history of my morning problem, and she was taking notes. After about ten minutes she stopped me, looked at me earnestly and said, 'Were you loved by your parents as a child?' I realised this was not for me. I couldn't get out of there fast enough, so I paid the bill and disappeared. It was like a sitcom special. Because my condition hadn't been apparent to them, it made me think, yet again, that I wasn't suffering anything of consequence. I left feeling I was just being stupid. I returned to doing what I had done for so long: telling myself to snap out of it. That it was mind over matter. That it was weakness.

'You can get on top of it.' That was what I had been telling myself for most of my life, because every day I did get on top of it. Often I would be saying it to myself in the most high-level meetings: Pull yourself together, just concentrate, get into this meeting. If I could get some adrenaline pumping, I would start to feel better. I knew I could still carry off the meeting, but I wouldn't be feeling confident. I would be acting, and that takes it out of you. People who have depressive conditions can become very practised at acting, but it is very frustrating. A similar meeting in the afternoon was completely different. There would be easy authority in my voice, a clarity in my thinking, a confidence. And I would enjoy myself.

So I knew I was experiencing this phenomenon that I had to deal with each morning. And I knew, as I grew older, it was dragging on later into the day. I had talked about it with Maureen, and I think subconsciously I knew I had a problem. It is very hard to admit that you've got depression. I was very conscious of the stigma attached to it. The combination of my background and being in public life meant I thought people would associate depression with weakness of character and so discount me from positions of great responsibility.

So there I was. I don't think I thought it through quite so consciously at the time, but I was very convinced that the 'depression label' could work strongly against me.

I spent five or six weeks agonising over this dilemma. In early July 2009 I flew to Washington and Beijing for a fortnight to get some idea of what the United States and China would do on climate change in the run-up to the Copenhagen global conference.

I had something like forty-four meetings during the two-week period, but I was by myself a lot outside the meetings. I had plenty of time to think, and I didn't feel well on many of those days. I was dealing with jet lag on top of it all, but on many days it wasn't until midmorning before I was snapping out of my morning funk. To help my mood I did my usual 1500-metre swim on most days, and I would go for a walk in the sunshine.

I had started swimming each day when I discovered I had high cholesterol aged forty-seven, and I felt that the exercise helped my moods. My older brother Christopher was staying with us in Sydney for a week when I was starting my swimming regime. Christopher has exercised seriously all his life, and he is full of beans in the morning. He'd come to wake me up at 6 a.m. to help get me into the routine. He told me later that the look on my face was like thunder and he thought I was going to thump him. We walked down to the Olympic Pool, next to the Sydney Harbour Bridge, with me mooching beside him—Christopher talking and me grunting. Likewise, I had also chanced upon the impact sunshine and sneezing has on the release of endorphins.

During my thirties and early forties we lived twenty minutes out of Canberra, at Wamboin. Canberra has more sunshine hours than the Gold Coast, even in winter. So on the drive in to work I would stop the car two or three times because I am one of those people who sneezes when looking at the sun. The subsequent endorphin rush would make me feel better, or at the very least the sunlight would help my mood.

In America I was swimming and walking if it was sunny, but I was not feeling good. It was not conducive to thinking about taking on more responsibility. Yet while I was in the United States and China, Malcolm Turnbull was at home announcing unilateral decisions about how we would ultimately support government legislation on an emissions trading scheme at the end of the year. It beggared belief and added to my sense that something needed to be done, or we would tear ourselves apart as a party.

I was disappointed because I had no plan to deal with my problem. I found in life that I could deal with lots of things—family crises, financial problems or whatever—as long as I had a strategy to extract myself or my family from the circumstance. But in this instance I was increasingly feeling that the morning problems were inhibiting me from doing properly what I already had on my plate, let alone higher responsibility. And I didn't have any game plan for trying to deal with it. There were lots of things I could do outside politics, but I had returned because I thought it was the profession to which I was best suited. I wanted to make the best contribution I could, and I thought I would have even more capability if I didn't have this black dog visiting me every morning.

When Tony Smith and others asked me directly about the leadership, I was interested but I couldn't shy away from 'the morning issue'. Trying to deal with it had become more invasive and more difficult. The trip to America and China only compounded my concerns as to whether I could try to challenge for the leadership, much less do the leader's job with whatever my condition was.

I came back and the chatter and speculation was still on. There were telephone conversations taking place. Another three or four people, including Peter Costello, rang asking if I would be interested in running if it turned out that Malcolm's leadership was terminal.

I would always say, 'Yes, I am interested and I'll give it some serious thought'. I believed I had a bit of breathing space because it usually takes time for that sort of assessment of a leader's position to properly emerge.

Later in the same month Peter Costello rang me again and said, 'Every way I look at this it's bad news for the party and bad news for Malcolm. I think it might be time for you to step up to the plate. So are you interested?'

I said, 'Yes I am, but I'll think about it'.

I was keen, very keen. It was an opportunity you may only get once and I thought I had the capacity in every other sense to make a fair fist of it. But I was worried that the morning problem was incompatible with the demands of leadership.

More than most others, I was well aware of what the leadership responsibilities would involve. In addition to being Campaign Director for the party in the 1993 and 1996 elections, I had also been Chief of Staff to Andrew Peacock in the 1990 election. Leadership of any political party is a 24/7 responsibility. Most days you need to be on your game from 5.30 a.m. until late into the night. The mornings are critical. I knew that if I gave the nod then many things would spin out of my control: you can be carried along by the support and the actions of others. You need to run with it, with no time for second thoughts. The last thing I wanted to do was begin something that I couldn't finish. Gnawing away in the back of my mind was the unspoken fear that I might let myself and others down if the black dog got in the way. It was time to seek professional assessment.

2

A PLAN'S THE THING

During the parliamentary winter break the phone calls continued. I was working in my electorate office, doing the usual round of meetings, and colleagues were still ringing to see if I had made up my mind.

Peter Costello even hinted that if I did contest and was successful, he might stay until the election to help me. It was a very generous offer and would have been influential in my decision if I had been well. I thanked him and said that if it was the end for Malcolm, then I was interested, and given what he had said, I would be thinking about it and taking his advice further.

As we were approaching the return to parliament in the second week of August, I knew crunch time was coming. Nothing had happened over recent weeks to allay my fears. If anything, my concerns were being compounded.

I confronted these worries during an interstate trip on 3 and 4 August. I was spending two days in rural Australia, something I would always look forward to, yet I really struggled through both days, only coming good in the evenings. I was visiting the South-West of Western Australia. My colleague in the seat of Forrest, Nola Marino, had organised a series of meetings with farming and mining interests. The round trip involved eight hours of flying time and four hours in a car. Time to think.

Did I really have a depressive condition? It was a hard reality to contemplate. On those flights I faced the fact that I had a problem. I decided that I was going to do something serious about it, and that I would do whatever it took to fix it, whatever the consequences.

I realised that if Malcolm fell over, there was no way I could seek to challenge him or compete against others if I was dealing with some sort of depression. It was the first time I accepted that there was a barrier to me going any further in my political career.

On my return home I discussed it with Maureen. I don't know if we had ever used the 'D' word. We had only talked about the creeping nature of my morning mood during my fifties. But I was blunt this time. I said, 'I've got a problem and I need to see a professional, a proper professional'. I had decided I would ring Jeff Kennett, the former Liberal premier who now headed beyondblue, an organisation providing information about depression. I still probably didn't say 'depression', I simply talked about 'my condition'.

Maureen was fine of course. She was probably relieved. We had been talking about the leadership issue and had both been worried about whether I could handle the job, because of my mornings.

I thought about what my father had said when I told my parents thirty-five years earlier that I was going to marry Maureen. He said, 'I don't know where you are heading son, but you are heading somewhere, and you have chosen someone very well equipped to go with you'.

The next day I spoke to my Victorian colleague, Tony Smith, who I had known for twenty years and with whom I had a frank and trusting relationship. I told him I was very keen to take up the challenge but that I had a problem that I needed to deal with first. I gave Tony a description of my condition and the conclusions that I'd reached. I told him that I was going to ring Jeff Kennett to seek his advice and a possible referral to somebody who could give me an opinion on what was going on, whether it was fixable and what I could do about it. Tony was understanding and supportive. He had high-flying friends who had dealt with depressive conditions successfully. On the Saturday morning I rang Jeff. He was driving out of Cradle Mountain with his wife Felicity on their way to a Hawthorn match in Launceston. The phone reception was poor. He said he would contact me when he got to the football oval. True to his word, at 1.30 p.m. Jeff rang and I gave him a rundown of my condition and symptoms, and explained why I was concerned about it at this stage with the question of the leadership on the table. Jeff understood the circumstances. I told him as much as I could about the politics and the pressure on me and that I needed to resolve it one way or another. I trusted him.

He said that he was no expert, but he would do what he could to find someone who could help me. He also said, 'Thank God you've confronted it'. He was reassuring, saying that half the battle is acknowledging the problem.

He rang again on early Monday morning, saying he had an eight o'clock appointment for me on Wednesday with Professor John Tiller, the distinguished psychiatrist at Melbourne University and the Albert Road Clinic in Melbourne. I was so grateful. I felt that someone was taking what I had told them seriously and doing something about it. I had made a start and, more importantly, I had a plan.

Professor Tiller said, 'Sit down and tell me about it'. He started taking notes. He was at his desk and I was in an armchair. These might be small things, but I felt better already because I wasn't on the stereotypical couch. I started talking, but he stopped me after about ten minutes and I thought, Oh God, here we go again, was I loved by my mother? But miraculously he said, 'Andrew, from what you've told me so far I just want to say to you this is fixable. You've got a chemical problem and this is fixable. Now go on'.

I talked for the next forty minutes, with him prompting and questioning me. He wanted the chronology of the condition and a bit of history about family members. It was as I imagined it should be, almost a businesslike discussion. He was interested in the facts.

He diagnosed diurnal variation, a condition that involves a daily variation of mood. In my case it meant that for the first two or three hours of each morning my mood was substantially different—almost the opposite of what it was for the remainder of the day.

Since my teenage years, I had found myself going to sleep taking on the world, being very positive about the issues that I was dealing with, identifying solutions to problems and planning how I might go about the next day's activities. I have never had a problem sleeping, no matter what political crisis was going on. When I woke six or seven hours later, I would instantly experience the same positive frame of mind that I had when I went to sleep, but it would only last a split second. It would then feel as though I was descending in an elevator, going down through different moods until I found myself in a highly negative state of mind, not wanting to turn on the radio, not wanting to get out of bed, not wanting to make decisions. Worst of all was knowing that this would be my lot for the next two to three hours.

Professor Tiller said the problem was fixable—that it was a chemical imbalance, a late release of serotonin—but he also told me that finding the solution might involve a lot of trial and error. He said having the condition for such a long time can lead to other psychological conditions, which might be best dealt with by a psychologist in due course. He also told me some people find that they can deal with such issues themselves once they have dealt with the underlying depressive illness. He was very open with me. It was a methodical and effective way of working through the issue.

He emphasised that psychiatry was not an exact science and that it could take a while to find the best chemical balance for me. He warned me that there could be significant and difficult short-term side effects to the treatments and that I couldn't expect any beneficial effect for four or five weeks at the earliest, or much longer perhaps. The side effects of the chemical cocktail would become apparent over that period of time.

Professor Tiller started me on Lexapro tablets that morning. He had clearly outlined the possible side effects for me, and there were many. There seemed to be about two-dozen possible reactions, from diarrhoea and putting on weight to skin conditions. One prominent side effect of Lexapro was that it could initially make you more depressed than the underlying condition. The label warned that someone around you should be alert to possible suicidal tendencies. But that was one of about twenty-four possible side effects; surely they were just covering themselves. Right?

Not only was I finally going to beat my morning funk (it even had a name!), but the timing suited the political demands on me. Four or five weeks to sort out the side effects meant that I could express interest in the leadership position, if it came to that, and be ready and well for the challenge, or the job.

I left the room ecstatic. It dawned on me as I travelled out to the airport to return to parliament that, for the first time in forty-three years, I might find myself free of this morning condition, and that I might be better than I'd ever been. It was an exhilarating moment. Above all, I had heard loud and clear, 'This is treatable'.

I flew back to Canberra that day. My phone rang while I was waiting in the lounge for my flight to be announced. It was Peter

Costello asking for my decision. I had not intended to tell too many people that I was under treatment, hoping to stay under the radar while I was finding a solution, coming out the other end to engage fully if Malcolm's leadership became untenable. Nevertheless, Peter was a special case. Despite being on the backbench, he was still, in practice, the most senior member of the Liberal parliamentary party, at least in Victoria, and he had intimated he would stay and assist me until the election if I was prepared to seek the leadership. I trusted him.

I told him about my circumstance and the outcome of the consultation, and that, without telling the world, I would find a solution over the coming weeks, experimenting with different medications, with the aim of being completely well within a few weeks. Peter was a bit taken aback, but sympathetic and encouraging. He was forensically enquiring into the nature of the condition and the name, and what it meant. I was so optimistic he said, 'OK, we'll just sit tight and see what happens', and he wished me good luck.

Of course, Professor Tiller's cautions went straight over my head. I was fixed on the fixable. Even speaking to Peter I was on a bit of a high, thinking I was on the road to recovery. I really thought I would pop a few pills and then have the medication sorted in a few weeks. It gave me time to re-engage with the leadership issues. I wouldn't need to tell many people and so would avoid the stigma attached to depression.

I only realise now how false these expectations were. I confronted my misplaced optimism at the first Shadow Cabinet meeting back in parliament. Shadow Cabinet meetings start with the Leader making political comments, followed by responses around the table. Godwin Grech was the backdrop to this meeting, as were Malcolm's subsequent climate change pronouncements. There was nothing challenging for me on the agenda and it was all a bit acrimonious.

Malcolm was chairing the meeting. I still hadn't come out of my morning malaise. I was negative, lacked confidence and didn't want to engage. I was sitting back in my seat, and Malcolm was just a couple of seats away from me. Whatever was being discussed, I didn't want to join in. People around the table were debating the issue and I just sat there feeling indecisive. My body language was submissive. All I could think was that there was absolutely no way I could be chairing this meeting. But half an hour later, sitting in the same meeting, which was by then even more testy, I was sitting there thinking, God I wish I was chairing this meeting.

The change was all in my head. All of a sudden I had clarity. Instead of thinking negative thoughts and that everything was too hard, all of a sudden a problem was an opportunity to do something. I was trying to catch the chairman's attention and was also busy writing notes to marshal my thoughts. I was listening earnestly to what people were saying to see whether I agreed or disagreed, and getting ready to respond. There was no lack of confidence anywhere within me. I argued my case. Robustly. Maybe even bullishly. I was enjoying myself. Leading the party? Why not?

But as I left the meeting room just after 11 a.m. there was just enough time to reflect on the previous hour. I had told myself all my adult life that I was not a morning person, but the starkness of that particular morning gave me an inescapable jolt. This couldn't be normal. It was a very strong affirmation of Professor Tiller's warning.

I had put up with fighting the morning problem for four decades, so how bad could any side effects be? Really bad, as it turns out. That first month on the tablets were the worst four weeks of my life.

3

GOING PUBLIC

During that first month when I was trialling the drugs, we had two sitting weeks. I was travelling a lot because it was two or three months from when the emissions trading scheme legislation was going to be presented to the House of Representatives again. We had voted against it the first time on my advice, and there was a lot of posturing about what would happen the next time.

As I was responsible for it, I had lots of meetings, press conferences, speeches, boardroom gatherings with CEOs and lunches where I was answering questions and explaining our position and concerns. At the same time I was discovering that the medication I was taking made me feel depressed 24/7.

I tried all the tricks I knew to make myself feel better. I arrived early at meetings so I could go for a walk in the sun. I told myself I was just unfortunate: I've got side effect number thirteen out of twenty-four, and it happens to be severe depression. I knew I had to put up with it for three or four weeks before my body adjusted.

I had never experienced anything like it. It was a lot worse than the underlying condition. It was a real hollowing out of yourself, not wanting to think about anything. At least in the past I knew I would slowly come out of it as the day progressed, but now I wasn't functioning well at any time of the day. I didn't want to make decisions, although I could force myself to, and I often spent hours looking at the wall in my office.

Vanessa Konig, my personal assistant, knew all the details and the impact the medication was having on me. Each morning she would ask how I was. 'I'm bad', was all I could say, and then I would just sit in my office with my door shut.

I had so much work to do, but I just couldn't bring myself to read. I avoided media, finding excuses, but there were many prior commitments I couldn't get out of. One of them was a speaking engagement at Birregurra, down in the Western District of Victoria, addressing about 250 farmers. For the complete trip I sat in the front of the car, with one of my staff members in the back, listening to classical music with my eyes closed. That always helped calm me.

The day had started with a press conference, followed by an Australian Industry Group lunch with fifteen CEOs. I had sat in the sun on a park bench for half an hour before the lunch meeting to try to give myself a lift. When I was meeting all the CEOs, I was feeling bad, lacking confidence. The adrenaline kicks in when I have to speak publicly, and it went very well, but afterwards I told my staff I had some things to do at home. Really, I just needed to sit in a chair. Later, they picked me up for Birregurra.

When we got there, everyone wanted to meet me because I used to run the National Farmers' Federation and it was a great social event. The local Country Women's Association had prepared the meal, and it was a typical rural bush evening, which I always enjoy. I was trying so hard to engage with everyone, but it was tough. Thankfully I was very much on top of the topic of the evening, climate change, and once I got to my feet the adrenaline surged.

There was an hour of questions and then everyone wanted to talk to me individually afterwards. I finally got back in the car at about 11.30 p.m. I was exhausted and it was a two-hour drive back to Melbourne. It was a pretty typical day, but with the depression everything was such an effort. I didn't want to talk on the way back, and I couldn't sleep, so again I just sat listening to classical music.

It was four weeks like that, just trying to keep lifting one foot after the other. It made me wonder about people who have chronic depression. What a curse.

Maureen's own recollection of those four weeks shows another perspective:

> When Andrew decides to do something, he gets on with it. He likes a plan of action, and Jeff Kennett facilitated that by recommending a psychiatrist who is of the same ilk. After the first visit to the psychiatrist, Andrew was quite buoyed up. This thing could be fixed and he was going to do it, and fast.
>
> Things did not go to plan. Chronic tiredness, listlessness, 24-hour depression, sleeplessness, jerking of his whole body when asleep and sweating all manifested themselves over the next three to four weeks. He had hardly told any-one what he was doing, so was trying to work and go about life as normal.
>
> Parliament was sitting in Canberra. Andrew had to travel from Canberra to Melbourne during the week a couple of times to see the psychiatrist. We are a close family and I would tell our children and parents or friends that he was coming back for a meeting. I knew our daughter was suspicious.
>
> The first lot of medication was a nightmare. It really drove him into deep depression. He was barely getting out

of bed. At least before starting the medication he would get out of bed, albeit very unwillingly. He would come home from work at three or four o'clock in the afternoon, unheard of for this workaholic. He would say that he couldn't do anything: not look at an email, not lift the phone, not read anything. He would just sit in his office looking at the walls. At home he would sleep on the couch with no interest in the news or anything else. Sleep at night was elusive, so he was taking sleeping tablets as well.

One of Andrew's sisters, Janet, and her husband Lindsay own a beach house at Aireys Inlet, so we asked if we could borrow it for a weekend. Andrew loves the beach, and a weekend like that is rare with his workload, so normally he would have been a pig in mud. Not this weekend.

I lit the open fire and Andrew lay on the couch and hardly moved or spoke for the weekend. He didn't want any television or music on. I looked after the fire and food and went for walks by myself. I persuaded him late on Saturday to come for a drive as there were some great houses to look at, something he would normally love. He looked at me as if I was asking him to go to the moon, but he came. I drove, pointing out houses and things that would usually interest him. He sat slumped in the passenger seat, barely saying a word. We left Aireys Inlet on Sunday afternoon, and I think it was the worst weekend either of us ever had.

I was worried that this medication was not going to work. The doctor had said that Andrew would probably get worse before he got better, and that lots of people did not stick it out. There is a very high percentage of people who give up the medication after only a few weeks. I had met the psychiatrist and had to be on suicide watch, so to

speak, because of the side effects of the medication. I think
I had been on duty all that weekend.

At the end of the four weeks, I had adjusted enough to the
medication, but the mornings were the same as they had always
been. Professor Tiller decided to double the dosage. He warned me
I could get the same side effects again.

The first day, a Friday, I didn't feel too bad, but I had to go back
to Canberra on the Sunday and I was cactus again. When I arrived in
Canberra at 8 p.m. on Sunday night I went straight to bed.

The next day, I was just going through the motions. There was a
Shadow Cabinet meeting, which I mumbled through. My vision of
getting on top of the condition, and the medication, within four to six
weeks was starting to explode.

People were still asking me about the leadership. I couldn't keep
saying, 'I'm thinking about it'. How long does one person need to
consider something like that? I realised I had to do something.
When Professor Tiller said I had to trial the increased dosage for
another month, I knew my timetable was shot. I didn't want to make
decisions, but I knew I couldn't put this one off for much longer.

On Tuesday morning there was the usual three-hour partyroom
meeting, which was held every week of parliamentary sittings. I was
really in a bad way. I listened for twenty minutes and then I saw the
sun shining outside, so I left.

It is probably a five-minute walk from the Liberal party room—
down a green-carpeted corridor, turn right, left and right again, and
out large glass doors, across the road that goes around Parliament
House—to some wonderful little gardens. It is not where you
would normally expect to find a senior member of the Coalition
during a partyroom meeting. They are very private gardens. There
are benches surrounded by rose bushes and wisteria hanging from
a pergola.

That is where I took myself at 9.15 a.m. on 15 September 2009, seeking respite from myself. I can only imagine what I looked like, sitting there alone on the bench with shoulders rounded forward. The sun was beating down, which made me feel better, and I didn't have to deal with anything. I could have stayed there for hours, but after fifty minutes my mobile phone rang. It was Nick Xerakias, my senior staff member. Malcolm had been in touch, wanting me back in the meeting. My stomach dropped. That was the last thing I wanted, but if the leader calls you, you go, no matter how you feel.

Normally the Shadow Cabinet members don't speak in the partyroom meetings, which can run for two or three hours. It's an opportunity for the party to go through the legislation that's coming up that week, to approve it or argue against it, and to raise any other issues on their minds. Shadow Cabinet brings recommendations, and Shadow ministers have to be on hand in case any backbench members want an explanation. There is also an hour or two where the backbenchers speak for up to five minutes on any topic, introduce an issue they're concerned about or inform the party about something. It can be political or policy. Shadow ministers can't speak unless by way of clarification. They've got the Shadow Cabinet meetings to debate issues. The partyroom meeting belongs to the backbenchers.

I didn't have any legislation that was coming up that week, so I had thought I would not be missed. The only reason that I would be called would be if something in my area had come up and Malcolm wanted me to deal with it. I trudged back feeling sorry for myself, not wanting to leave the sun, and wondering what it was all about.

Entering the party room, I was hit with someone in full swing attacking Malcolm's implied support for the government's emissions trading scheme. The idea of having to form a view, to respond quickly, just felt like an impossible effort. The adrenaline always gave me a rush but invariably not until I got to my feet.

Malcolm said, 'Oh well, Andrew's back now'. He said there were four or five more members who wanted to speak on the topic and that I would then have to sum up. That gave me time to find out what everyone was concerned about and formulate a response. Basically, it was an attack on Malcolm's position on the government's climate change legislation. Technically, we had not made any decisions about how we would deal with the second lot of emissions trading scheme legislation, and we had a process we were supposed to be going through to arrive at a position. But everyone was conscious that Malcolm had, on several occasions, intimated that at the end of the day we'd cave in to whatever the government presented. That's what everyone was upset about. Backbenchers are not bashful: they say what's on their mind, and some think they've got nothing to lose because they feel that under a particular leader they're never going to get promoted anyway. These issues are always a backdrop.

The four or five speakers went for it in quite an aggressive way. I had started coaching myself: get ready to stand up, listen, make some notes. Usually I would be taking lots of notes, but all I could manage was four lines, four propositions. And then Malcolm called on me. All that time I was just wishing for the floor to open up so I could disappear through it.

I forced myself to stand up, I started walking towards the front of the room and then it happened. The adrenaline started pumping, my thoughts came together, and I argued coherently for ten minutes. I dealt with the issue without slighting Malcolm, and reassured everyone there was a process we were going to follow. I gave them a sense that they were still in control and that Malcolm would be part of that process. I can't really remember what I said, but whatever it was seemed to reassure everyone, and it was said with enough conviction and authority that it was effective. It shut the issue down for Malcolm, at least for that meeting. I sat down.

Peter Costello was in the room. We hadn't seen each other for a few weeks, and he must have thought, Oh, Robbie's back in action. He wasn't alone. My speech, or rather my performance, prompted two or three of the people who had been encouraging me to run for the leadership, people with influence over different blocks of members, to think they should get in touch with me again.

Of course, they didn't know that a few minutes after sitting down I was back in the black again. I left the meeting. I was feeling really bad again and I went back to my office, said to Vanessa, 'I'm feeling crap. I don't want to see anyone', closed the door and sat watching the wall.

That's what I was doing when Peter called half an hour later. He's got such a big, booming voice and he sounded excited. 'Robbie, what's happening?' he said. Clearly he thought I had found the magic chemical cocktail, that I was on my way back, ready to engage. 'Mate', I answered, 'I have never felt so bad in all my life'.

What could he say? He'd just seen me performing really well and he was thinking I was on my way, that things might be shifting. Peter was clearly taken aback, and could only utter, 'Fair enough. Get well'. (A couple of weeks later he would declare that he was pulling up stumps and leaving, twelve months before the expected timing of the election.)

There was no plan B. Everyone was very disillusioned with Malcolm. Tony Abbott and Joe Hockey aspired to the job but thought they needed more time to position themselves better.

Later that morning, I got another two or three calls from people asking me if I had made up my mind. I said, 'I'm still thinking about it, but I will give you an answer shortly', because I knew I was starting to look stupid.

By then it was about noon and I realised I wasn't going to resolve the medication issue quickly. I decided I had no alternative but to seek some space. The only way that was going to happen was by leaving the Shadow Cabinet, and to do that I had to give a reason. The last thing I wanted to do was be dishonest, so I had to weigh up the consequences.

I still hadn't told my three kids, any of the other staff, most of my work colleagues, my parents … yet I was in a better frame of mind because I was starting to formulate a plan. I knew I had to take some action. I was just going through all the permutations and combinations and consequences, but I knew the critical thing was going public. All the rest would fall into place.

It would give me the freedom to deal with the side effects. People would understand that I wasn't well. And I wanted to retain my integrity. I needed to be honest with people. I think it's a lot easier for everybody if you tell them what's going on. It was complicated in this case because there's a stigma attached to depression and I was very conscious of the conventional wisdom—that a mental disorder is seen as a character weakness—and politically that it could mitigate against me, no matter how well I recovered. But I couldn't be cowered by that.

I decided I didn't care. I had nothing to prove. I was holding myself hostage to my own ambitions. I came to the conclusion that the most important thing was beating the depression. How good would that be? And my example might just help other people who thought as I had for so long. Potentially I could feel better than I ever had before, and if it meant the end of my political career, then I knew there were still a thousand things I could do outside of politics. (As it turned out, the first week I did go public I had two major job offers, so that was encouraging.)

I arranged to see Malcolm at 8.30 p.m. that night and told him everything. He was very good about it, as I expected he would be. I have known him a long time and he's a decent fellow. We agreed I would take leave until Christmas from the Shadow Cabinet but stay in the parliament doing my electorate work. It gave me control over my agenda. I thought Ian Macfarlane was best placed to take over the climate change portfolio, and Malcolm spoke to him later that night.

Then I rang Laurie Oakes and arranged to meet him the next day. I wanted to see if he would consider writing a column. Laurie has a big following across Australia in major News Limited weekend papers with huge circulations, and he is one of the most senior political journalists in the country. He's highly respected, and I believed he was the best journalist for the job. I wanted to get the story out with some sort of history and context, as I didn't want people thinking I was in a foetal position under the table. I thought Laurie would do a much better job writing the story than I could.

I was still determined to get well and then perform at a more senior level. I wanted to show that I could have a condition like this and beat it. Laurie and I spoke for an hour on the Wednesday, and he sent me a copy of the article on Friday, which he normally wouldn't do. I was very impressed by the piece, and touched by how sensitively he treated the issue.

I travelled to Melbourne and called in unannounced to see my parents, Marie and Frank, in Reservoir on the Friday morning. I told them everything and explained that there would be an article about it the next day in the *Herald Sun*. They are in their eighties and have nine kids and thirty-four grandchildren, so not much surprises them, but this took them a little unawares.

Except for my early years, I had always been quiet in the mornings, and although I hadn't lived at home much since I was seventeen, they could see I had acted in a way that was consistent with what I was saying. My mother said I had been the happiest of all their nine children during childhood but had gone quiet in the mornings in my teens. They had put it down to the impact of adolescent hormones.

When I had the copy of the article on the Friday night, I sent it to my three kids with a little note. I then rang them. Tom was living in London at the time. I hadn't wanted to bother or worry them about it before. I also sent copies to my parents and my brothers and sisters, and rang Christopher, who then contacted my other siblings.

Maureen was relieved. She contacted her sister and brother to let them and their families know what was happening. She had said very little to anyone, often covering for me over the preceding weeks, saying I had the flu and couldn't shake it.

I was still struggling with the depression, but I had instituted an action plan, and I knew I was going to be in control of commitments come Saturday. I wasn't feeling trapped, and I always knew I was suffering side effects. At the very least I knew I could go back to the way I had been, just dealing with it in the morning rather than all day.

When Laurie's column came out, Nick Xerakias referred publicity enquiries back to the News Limited article. TV stations had existing footage of me, so people could see I wasn't in a totally debilitated state. That was the beauty of going public in this way. I avoided looking as though I was making a meal of this yet had a hand in how the story had been told.

Neil Mitchell was chasing me for an interview, and I decided I would do one live interview and leave it at that. People could then refer to either the column or the interview. Monday morning the adrenaline was coursing when I was on air, so I felt good. The message got out quickly and effectively. It was important that I let the people in my electorate know. I have nearly 700 party members in my electorate, and it was vital that they had a clear idea of what was going on. Once I had done the interviews for the column and the radio, that was it. I didn't want to do anything else until I had found an answer.

A lot of people were surprised. I am not the most gregarious sort of character; I am sociable but I am not the life of the party, and a lot of people are a bit quiet in the mornings anyway, for all sorts of reasons. So people were taken aback by the extent of what I described.

Parliament sat the subsequent week. I was fine while I was working in my electorate and providing help to Ian Macfarlane, which I did for three or four weeks. But in parliament I felt redundant. I wasn't feeling good because of the medication, and I felt I had nothing to contribute. Everyone was telling me to rest, so I thought I should just go away. I didn't feel like resting because not having to deal with the media or all the speaking engagements already felt like a holiday.

But Maureen and I decided to go to Blue Bay on the New South Wales central coast for two weeks. We rented a great place right on the rocks at the water's edge. Friends and our children visited; the weather was good and I was thinking that it should be fantastic— the sun, the water, no responsibilities—but I was just so depressed. I read some detective novels and I ploughed through the second *Underbelly* series. It was better than sitting up in parliament feeling the way I did, but it was still pretty bad. I was conscious of what was happening; I wasn't defeatist. I felt I had to put up with the state of mind, the side effects, get through it and see what happened next.

But in the end nothing happened next. We got back from the beach and the all-day depression improved, but there was no change in the morning state of mind. It was time to rethink the medication.

4

GETTING A BALANCE

I returned to my electorate. I was moping around wondering every day if that would be the day the drugs started working. Each time I walked into the office, all my staff would ask 'How are you feeling this morning?'

'No different', I would have to answer. It was a daily ritual.

It wasn't a good time for Maureen. She was quite worried. I was depressed and couldn't muster any enthusiasm or interest in anything. I never got to the stage of feeling suicidal though, as warned in the medication instructions. The one saving grace was that, whenever I felt really down, I would remind myself that the day-in-day-out depression was a side effect of the drug. I never contemplated stopping the medication, because it had a purpose. I wanted to get better, but I needed space to do that. That's why I went public. Even if it took me twelve months, I was going to persist until we found an answer. I had great confidence in what Professor Tiller had said.

Happily, I didn't lose my appetite or my taste for a glass of wine or a Scotch. It had just been a bad patch. I did worry though about having gone public and whether I would ever be able to return to politics effectively.

Professor Tiller took me off Lexapro and started me on a desvenlafaxine-based drug called Pristiq. The first morning after the first dose I felt better than I had for months. My spirits jumped. Sadly it didn't last, but at least it didn't make me depressed 24/7. This drug made me very tired for much of the day. I'd be catching ten-minute catnaps whenever I could.

The initial positive response kept me and Professor Tiller interested. Yet persistence was the order of the day. The dosage levels were increased regularly, with occasional positive days soon after each increase, but in the end nothing happened for months, despite the daily dosage going from 50 mg to 100 mg, 150 mg … 200 mg. But I know other people who have had to experiment for very much longer.

By the time Professor Tiller gave me the option of 250 mg or 300 mg, I thought, bugger it, let's get on with it. So in March 2010, I increased the dosage to 300 mg. I had a good day the next day, then a couple of days when I was better than I had been since starting the new drug. Then days of being better than I could ever remember.

I didn't like to say anything—I was worried it could all change—but I started to say to my staff, 'I'm feeling maybe a bit better'. I waxed and waned like that for a week. The tiredness hung around for a while, but the morning fog just vanished.

I found myself in the bathroom at 5.45 a.m. each morning just marvelling at how clear-headed and positive I was. It was life-changing stuff. My morning swim in Port Philip Bay was taking me nearly one and a half hours, instead of just one, because I was initiating conversations with everybody. Maureen would get up while I was swimming and find all the daily papers already read and the *Today Show* blaring along with the radio. It was a first in thirty-five years of marriage.

The previous November, Professor Tiller had started talking about a broad range of treatments to help me. He said herbal medicine or acupuncture assisted some people. He thought it was important to investigate the relationship that biorhythms might be having on my mental disposition. It was an emerging science, he said, but one we should try because medication alone was often not the complete answer.

While I was still experimenting with different levels of Pristiq, Professor Tiller referred me to Dr David Cunnington, a sleep-disorders physician. I've never had a problem sleeping. It's how I have felt when I have woken up that's been the problem.

A lot of people—shift workers, young people—are vulnerable to their normal biorhythms being disturbed. It can lead to their bodies producing serotonin, melatonin and other chemicals at the wrong time, greatly affecting their normal sleep patterns and/or mood.

To get some idea of what was going on, Dr Cunnington gave me an electronic pill, which took two days to pass through me. At the same time he strapped a receiver to my chest, and for the next two days the pill transmitted my core body temperature every ten seconds. He then graphed the two days of recorded temperatures. 'There's your problem', he said, pointing to the two mornings where my core body temperature hit a minimum at 6 a.m. He explained that when your core body temperature hits its low, a message is sent to your brain telling it to stop producing melatonin and start producing serotonin. Most people's core body temperature hits a minimum between 2 a.m. and 3 a.m.; mine was three or four hours later. Cunnington explained that for the first three or four hours of my waking day I had much less serotonin than I should, and this could significantly affect my mood. He said for people like me, this period of serotonin deficiency was often associated with a depressive condition, which could extend as a person aged. It meant that when I was waking up at 6 a.m. I was probably feeling the same as other people would feel if they were consistently woken up at 2 a.m. Bingo.

For the first time I could make some sense of my morning problem, and why I had popped out of it, initially at about 8 a.m. and in my later years at 9 a.m., 10 a.m. or even noon. Again, unlike others, at least I popped out of it each day.

Scientists still don't understand it well, but our bodies fill with melatonin at night, and this has a relationship to how much serotonin you then produce to fire you up for the day ahead. Depressed people generally have quite low levels of melatonin. Why? Again it's not known.

In consultation with Professor Tiller, Cunnington put me on a melatonin tablet at night, and the Pristiq medication also encouraged the production of serotonin during the last few hours of the night. It meant that when I woke, I should have appropriate levels of melatonin and serotonin to make me feel normal.

Dr Cunnington also added a further stimulus to serotonin production. There are cells in your eyes that have the sole function of identifying morning daylight and sending a signal to your brain to start producing serotonin. It is the blue part of the light spectrum that performs these tricks, and it can penetrate your closed eyelids (just as when you look at a bright light with your eyes closed, you can see brightness). It's why many people feel better if they sleep with the curtains open. There is a portable, rechargeable panel of blue light available (about the size of a square CD holder) that I carry whenever I am travelling. It is too bright to look at directly, but I put it at an angle to shine across my eyes every morning at 6 a.m. while I read the papers: more serotonin prompting. I am leaving nothing to chance!

The aim of the blue light and the melatonin tablet is to reset my sleep/wake cycle so that I might reach a minimum body temperature earlier in the night—closer to 2 a.m. rather than 6 a.m.

Because I have had my problem since my teenage years, it is unlikely my cycle will change greatly; it is now hardwired in my system. These strategies can usually alter the sleep/wake cycle for a shift worker in three or four days. It is clearly going to take a little longer for me.

Professor Tiller said many depressive conditions begin with a trauma or a succession of traumas that, for some reason, block the release of the chemicals necessary for normal mental health. Looking back, I wonder whether leaving the family farm and dealing with years 7 and 8 of school triggered this sort of response in my body. My mother certainly suspects that may be the case, given my disposition in the morning before and after that period.

5

WHEN MORNINGS WERE BRIGHT

It snowed the night I was born. It was as unusual then as it would be today. My parents, Frank and Marie, lived on a lovely sheep property at Flowerdale, a hamlet an hour and half north of Melbourne in the Great Dividing Range. That night in August 1951, my father drove my mother slowly through the falling snowflakes to the Mercy Hospital in East Melbourne in a truck.

I was only four when we left Flowerdale, but I can clearly remember shearing time there: my father would be bent over sheep after sheep. I would be allowed to visit with my mother and Christopher when we took morning or afternoon tea. Even today, I still love the smell of shearing sheds.

Despite it being the time of the wool boom and therefore a profitable time to be a sheep farmer, my parents' educational ambitions for their four children (and more were planned) prompted them to sell up and move closer to the best schools they hoped one day to be able to afford. This was a constant: our parents always urged us to make the most of educational opportunities.

For nine months we lived at nearby Yea after the sale of the Flowerdale property while we were searching for a new home. During World War II, my two sets of grandparents had owned cafes on opposite sides of Yea's main street. It was in Yea that my parents had met, in the years following the end of the war. Because I hadn't yet started school, I often went with my father when he did a bread run to the farms in the surrounding districts. The smell of freshly baked bread filled the van. That magical bread smell is my abiding memory of those few months.

My parents bought a dairy farm 5 kilometres north of Epping, on the outskirts of Melbourne. The farm was delivering milk under contract to the Melbourne milk market. In those days the milk was transported in the old milk cans. In the mid-1950s, Epping was a country town. It had a general store, a petrol station, a pub, a milk bar, a butcher, the council chambers and probably fifty to sixty homes.

I started school at St Peter's Primary in Epping, run by the Good Samaritan nuns. Life was dominated by sport and the farm. For six months of the year, I went to sleep dreaming of kicking the winning goal for the 'mighty' Demons (Melbourne Football Club) in the then VFL, and during the warmer months I could only think of cricket or riding our first pony, a white Welsh mountain mare named Gay Lady. I loved that horse. My ambition was to be a jockey, but as I outgrew that possibility, I settled for being a farmer and a VFL footballer.

During those years, I always felt that we were privileged and well off, largely, I think, because so many other kids and primary-school classmates—all of whom came from the suburbs of Lalor or Thomastown—were always so keen to visit or spend weekends with us and just do what we were doing: checking the rabbit traps, helping with the milking, kicking the footy, riding a horse, exploring the hills, swimming in the creek or the dams, riding some of the sheep on the neighbours' property, smoking in the hay shed or bringing the cows in.

We were well fed and well loved, and it was a happy household. We often had picnics up past Kinglake on the King Parrot River or visited grandparents, and we went regularly to see the Epping Football Club, the 'Pings', play in the Diamond Valley Football League. Christopher and I would have a sarsaparilla soft drink on the footpath outside the Epping pub afterwards, while Dad had a beer or two before heading home to milk the cows.

I took it for granted that fathers worked seven days a week, and for the seven years we were at the dairy farm, my father didn't miss a milking, morning or night! My parents never burdened us with any of the financial difficulties they must have had in caring for us. By the time we left the farm seven years later, I had six siblings: Christopher, Janet, Beth, Carmel, Peter and Mary. Bernard and Helen arrived later, in Reservoir.

It was a tough time when our paddocks were completely burnt. The house, sheds and the cows were saved, but very sadly a neighbour died trying to get through our fence to fight the fire. His knapsack got caught in the fence and the fire overran him, burning him beyond recognition. Initially the locals who discovered him thought it was my father. I remember watching the smoke billowing over the hills and my parents loading us into our FJ Holden and filling the boot with all our memorabilia. Mum drove us away while dad stayed to save the cows. I felt excitement and fear, but we kids felt we were safe as long as our parents were taking control of the situation.

Nearly thirty years later, I had the same experience when Maureen, our three children, Tom, Joe and Pip, and our two dogs, Bassey and Beau, had to leave our property at Wamboin, 20 kilometres east of Canberra, as a deliberately lit fire swept across the valley below, heading directly for the steep ridge where we lived. Again, all our property, comprising 30 acres of wonderful ghost gums, was burnt, but the fire spared our house and horse, Nightmare (she was a very black mare!), whom I'd left feeding on a bale of lucerne hay at the back of the house.

My parents took a heavy and cruel financial blow in the aftermath of their fire in 1959, roughly midway through the 1957–60 drought. If some locals hadn't saved 1500 bales of our hay reserves, and my father hadn't ridden through the flames on his horse Smokey to save the milking cows, things would have been catastrophic.

As it was, during one subsequent month, the cows' milk production fell short of the contracted amount by 4 or 5 gallons a day. The milk company, Metropolitan Dairies in Gilbert Road, West Preston, cut my father's contract by 12 per cent. No leeway was given for getting burnt out. It meant that my parents were getting 2 per cent return on their investment, not enough to feed and educate their seven kids. (This precipitated our move to the suburbs three years later in 1963.)

I developed a great love of the land during those years. We were surrounded by hills and open paddocks and wonderful rock outcrops, a product of now extinct volcanoes from many centuries ago. For years—occasionally with Christopher but more often with my sister Janet—I would explore the hills and the creeks, taking in the views, sitting in the bush and listening to birds, skinny dipping in the creek and watching out for snakes.

I would have a great sense of anticipation when I got up early on a frosty morning before anyone else (apart from my father) to check if I had caught some rabbits in the many traps I used to lay. After watching my father set traps and recover rabbits, I thought I was ready to go it alone, but catching my first rabbit was a traumatic experience and affected me for the rest of my life. I set a number of traps half a mile from the house down near the local creek and went to bed full of expectation. I got up early and, very nervously, made my way down through the paddocks, through a light fog and an eerie silence. The first two or three traps were as I'd left them, then I came over a little knoll and my heart missed a beat as I saw a fully grown, live rabbit caught in one of the traps.

I spent a good ten minutes surveying the scene, preparing myself to wring the rabbit's neck as I had watched my father do on many occasions and thinking how I would proudly take my bounty home. All the while the rabbit was eyeing me off. I finally confronted the poor rabbit and tried to replicate the way my father would have killed it. Without strength or technique, I realised after ten minutes of awful struggle that I wasn't going to succeed, so I decided the only thing I could do was to cut its throat and put it out of its misery. I had my trusty pocketknife, but as it wasn't very sharp, I only succeeded after the sun was well up and the fog had cleared.

The elation of catching my first rabbit was severely dulled by my sense of guilt over the manner in which the animal had died. It distressed me greatly, and I decided never to put any animal through any unnecessary pain and suffering in the future. I got my father to show me how to efficiently and quickly wring a rabbit's neck, and I became quite proficient at catching them, which did contribute to family meals. I still hunger for my mother's wonderful rabbit stew.

I had a similar experience with birds. Christopher and I had air rifles, which we initially aimed at targets, but then we started shooting at sparrows and other small birds. One Saturday morning I spotted a sparrow high up in one of the trees. I took aim and fired, and the sparrow, to my surprise, dropped and landed a few feet in front of me. Picking it up, I saw what a beautiful little thing it was as it died in my hand. For the first time I felt a sense of shame for needlessly shooting such a wonderful creature. So, at age ten, I decided never to shoot birds for sport again, drawing a clear distinction between killing animals for food and pursuing them for sport.

Unfortunately, the three dogs I owned during those dairy-farm years didn't come to learn the same lesson. They doubled as pets for me and cow herders for my father. After I'd had my first dog, Blacky, for slightly more than a year, I came home from school one day to be told by my father, 'Son, I've had to take your dog Blacky down to the gully'. I soon realised that was a euphemism for having to shoot my dog. Blacky had been maiming the chooks, a habit from which a dog can't be broken. I didn't want to subject our many chooks to that after my experience with the rabbit, and my sadness was tempered by the promise of a new pup.

The new pup and I were great friends, and my father trained the dog to bring in the cows in the morning and afternoon, but a year or so later I came home from school again to be told, 'Son, I am sorry but I've had to take your dog Freddie down to the gully'. Freddie had been killing the neighbour's lambs.

I was learning about life on the land the hard way. The sadness was again tempered by my father promising to get me another pup, Charlie, who proved to have no vices and grew to be a reasonably effective cattle dog. When we ultimately left the dairy farm to settle in suburban Reservoir, my parents broke the news that it was no place for a cattle dog. Again I was broken-hearted and spent many days talking to Charlie about the injustice of it all.

Nevertheless, Charlie was one of the items available at our clearing sale before we headed off to the city. To my disbelief, he sold for five pounds, which seemed like a small fortune to me. I had a few words with the new owner and he seemed to me to be a good bloke with lots of cattle that needed rounding up, so I consoled myself with the thought that Charlie was doing what he liked best and that I'd been well remunerated for my loss.

Our parents demonstrated a remarkable work ethic over those seven years on the dairy farm. It left a deep impression on me and my siblings. They didn't have the finances to employ someone to help with the milking, and my mother was dealing with a bunch of kids.

They shouldered their responsibilities gladly and willingly, and never burdened their kids with things that we could do nothing about. It was a great example for all of us to take into adulthood and our own experience as parents.

Helping my father in the milking shed, I got an insight into a character trait that I certainly inherited. It takes a lot to get my father to lose his temper, but when he does, it's full on. One day, one of our bulls found its way into a paddock of maize that was ready for harvesting. After the milking was done, my father and I went down to get the bull out of the paddock, but after 45 minutes all we had to show for our efforts was a field of half-trampled crop. My father had had enough. He marched up to the house, grabbed his double-barrel shotgun, loaded it, marched back to the paddock, lined the bull up and shot both barrels into it's backside from 30 metres. The bull never stopped running until it had charged through three fences and into the neighbour's property. I share some of this trait. It takes a lot for me to lose my temper, but when I do, I invariably say or do things that I have sometimes regretted. I work hard to keep a lid on it.

Those pre-teenage years spent on a farm dealing with animals, fires, floods, disease and death introduced me to many experiences that have stood me in good stead. One of these experiences involved our pony, Gay Lady, and her foal. My sister Janet and I, aged eight and six and a half, especially loved that horse and spent hours riding her bareback, often double dinking. So when she was in foal, the sense of anticipation was immense. It was the start of the Gay Lady dynasty.

I love everything about horses: the smell, the independence, the arrogance, the strength and the sense of friendship once you've gained their trust. I have never lost the love of horses and have owned horses for much of my life, even trying my hand at polocrosse (the poor man's polo) for a period in the 1990s. When I go to the races, I spend most of my day at the mounting yards, just marvelling at the wonderful animals.

The foal had strong chestnut markings, a proud if somewhat uncertain bearing and a wonderful face. It was only some hours after this newborn foal found his feet that he started to circle, and so it was for the next couple of days—he would spend the day going around and around in circles. The vet was called and we discovered the foal had a blocked bowel. Once that was cleared, he had his first substantial drink from his mother, and we all went to bed thinking that all was well with the world and our new foal was now healthy and raring to go.

The next morning was a Saturday. I rose early and darted outside and down into the horse paddock. Gay Lady was standing over a dead foal. It turned out that two days without milk followed by a big drink and other complications had led to his death overnight. It was my first taste of the death of something loved. I spent much of the day, traumatised, in my favourite tree trying to reconcile the death of this much-longed-for foal.

Dad dug a hole in the horse paddock, and we gave the foal a decent burial. I was sad for some weeks, but it no doubt hardened me further for the ebb and flow of life. It also taught me another important lesson: nothing, good or bad, is ever over until it's over. I know that to be true in business and politics: no deal is ever done until it's truly done. No agreement is ever sealed until it's signed. No political contest is ever certain until the vote. My experience with that foal taught me not to make assumptions about success, to keep the pressure on until the bitter end, to stay alert always to what could go wrong before things are truly finalised.

When we moved to Reservoir, we gave Gay Lady to a large family from Epping. It was decades later that I learnt that Gay Lady had subsequently had two magnificent foals. My parents had kept it from me so as not to disappoint me.

It was at St Peter's that I was first introduced to power and politics—in the school yard. Perhaps being called 'wog' every day made Aldo, a big, athletic fellow in my class, angry, but he was the feared leader in the playground. After inadvertently giving him some lip one day, I found myself on the ground being thrashed. From then on, Aldo took every opportunity to line me up when we were playing football or to seek to provoke me in different ways.

I decided I needed a strategy to neutralise his growing influence in my life, and I noticed that he never took on Freddie Hanlon, a big boy with a sense of confidence and entitlement, perhaps because his father and uncle were (and still are) well-known and respected members of the racing fraternity. I made a point of getting to know Freddie a lot better, and with our shared rural backgrounds and interest in horses, we formed a friendship.

From that time onwards, whenever it looked like I was about to have trouble with Aldo, Freddie would appear and all was good. It was probably my first experience of the interplay of power, and of the benefit of forming coalitions.

Religion played a big part in my childhood. The priests and the nuns at the school had a great sense of authority about them, and it gave a great stability and certainty to so much of our lives. Everything was seen very much in black and white terms, and mostly the nuns and the teachers at St Peter's reinforced the values to which our parents strongly adhered—namely, the importance of respect and concern for one another, taking responsibility for your own actions, making the most of the talents you'd been given, love, family, friendships and hard work.

In the main, the nuns were a pretty good bunch, dedicated to their profession and capable teachers, but there were exceptions, and the dwindling numbers of young women seeking a vocation meant that many of the older nuns were staying on as teachers well beyond a sensible retirement age.

This was true of Mother Columbkille, who taught a combined years 7 and 8 class. She was a terror who employed all sorts of punishments to encourage our attention and learning. If you were sitting at your desk, it was not unusual to have her come from behind and wrap you over the knuckles with the metal side of the ruler, or punch you in the shoulder blade or arm.

It was probably a good character-forming experience, but it meant I didn't particularly enjoy school and sometimes felt frightened and angered by her behaviour. But I didn't dream of telling my parents, except for the time when she thumped the scab from my tuberculosis injection. My shirt sleeve under my jumper was drenched in blood from top to bottom, and it was my birthday. When I got home, I burst into tears.

She was perhaps most famous for ordering students to write answers on the board, and if the answer was not correct, Mother Columbkille would grab a handful of your hair and bang your face into the board. This was too much for one of the lads in Year 8. A number of the boys were marking time until they were old enough to go out and work; a couple of them were already shaving, and they could be physically intimidating. This didn't deter Mother Columbkille. After struggling to get a correct answer from one boy, she started to rub his face into the board; he turned and dropped Mother Columbkille where she stood.

The culprit was expelled, along with two or three of his mates who had urged him on. The class received a talking to from the priest and the deputy principal. Mother Columbkille returned somewhat subdued, yet within a fortnight she was back to her old terrorising self. I have never found anybody on the other side of the chamber or on the other side of the business desk—with the exception perhaps of Kerry Packer—who could create anywhere near that level of apprehension.

Was it then that I started feeling anxious in the mornings? I wonder. I would have had good reason to. It was the same year that we moved to Reservoir, though I continued Year 7 at Epping by catching the train. I felt a great sense of loss leaving the farm, and I was dealing with a fearful teacher at St Peter's.

My maternal grandparents, Fred (Pop) and Margaret Summers, had fascinating lives. They got married in their very early twenties, with Fred working in the sawmills at Yarck, a little town on the way to Mansfield. Aged twenty-one, Fred strained his heart working in the mills, a condition that affected him throughout his life. With a weakened heart, Fred took some years to properly recuperate and, in the meantime, had to find employment that was far less physical. It turned out Fred was a born salesman and trader, and he and my grandmother ultimately made a great success of their cafe in the main street of Yea.

I got to know them well as a child, when they had a dry-cleaning and baby clothes business in Sydney Road, Coburg, one of Melbourne's more multicultural suburbs, where they lived on top of and behind the shop. They also owned a lovely property at Kerrisdale, a small district on the road between Yea and Seymour just over the divide in north-east Victoria. I loved visiting both places. At the dry-cleaners I was always fascinated by the many different types of people who came and went. My grandmother was a great conversationalist, and Christopher, Janet, Beth and I were introduced to so many people, from so many different ethnic backgrounds, who chatted with my grandmother.

This continued my introduction to the diversity of Australia's postwar migrant experience. My primary school had many Italians and some Greeks, whose families had moved into the then new outlying suburbs of Lalor and Thomastown. Reservoir was similar. Coburg was a great melting pot. I suspect my early interest in and exposure to the different motivations and perspectives of the myriad groups that make up our community explain my ultimate attraction to politics, where every day you are charged with trying to reconcile hundreds, if not thousands, of competing and legitimate interests. That is at the heart of our job.

Of course, like all good grandmothers, Nan had an endless source of lollies. She also had the most outstanding passionfruit vine out the back of the shop. This was a fruit we hadn't known until they bought the shop, but we made up for lost time.

My abiding memory of that shop was going to sleep at nights in the upstairs bedroom, which fronted on to Sydney Road, and the trams rumbling by. For some reason I got a great sense of peace listening to the unique rhythm and sounds of the trams as they travelled up and down.

It probably explains my practice of the last few decades of going to sleep listening to some of the great Gregorian chants or the music of other wonderful choirs, such as those of King's College, Cambridge or Corpus Christi. Despite my love of jazz, my favourite piece of music is the *Miserere*.

The farm at Kerrisdale opened up another world to me. It was there that I was first introduced to an illegal act by Pop, on the property's mile-long frontage to the Goulburn River. Every time we visited, my grandfather would take Christopher and me down to the river to a quiet spot and proceed to pull in the drum net, a simple structure made with wire netting in the shape and size of an old 44-gallon drum, with an opening that fish can find their way into but can't find their way back out of.

The Goulburn River was rich with all sorts of fish and the occasional water rat and eel. Freddie Summers caught them all. I don't think there was an occasion when we pulled in the drum net and didn't find it half full of many different types of fish, almost all of which I'd never seen before.

It was all very exciting and spoilt me for life as far as fishing is concerned. I haven't got a lot of patience at the best of times, but having been introduced to fishing with a drum net, it's been very hard ever since to put in the long hours with the line and hook. Of course, it was illegal, but keeping an eye out for the possible appearance of a ranger added immeasurably to the excitement. In any event I always had great confidence that my silver-tongued grandfather—who finished up as the land sales manager with Victorian Producers— would talk his way out of it.

6

UPHEAVAL

The start of secondary school coincided with significant changes. We had moved from the farm at Epping midway through 1963 to a big weatherboard house on a large block in the northern suburb of Reservoir. At that time, thousands of acres of farmland were being progressively turned into suburban estates; our house was part of that development.

Reservoir was home to many immigrants, mainly Italians and some Greeks, who came to Australia after the war. Since then, some members of every wave of immigration have found their way to Reservoir: Indochinese, Eastern Europeans, Sri Lankans, Indians and, more recently, Africans, Iraqis and Afghanis.

My parents still live in Reservoir but are now in a retirement village looking down over Latrobe University and out to the hills of the Great Divide. Australia's successful postwar immigration experience is evident on the occasions I go with my parents to mass at St Gabriel's, Reservoir. The congregation, an eclectic group of people from so many nations, is always an inspiration and a source of pride for me. From jet-black Africans to the lily-white Irish, all are satisfying their spiritual needs and meeting as a community under one roof.

I had deeply loved the farm and was distressed when we left, but I slowly warmed to the experiences and opportunities offered by city life. After a lifetime of moving, I know I am the sort of person who can live anywhere, at least for a year or two. I have fond memories of every experience, but each time we move I now find myself looking forward to the unknown.

This attitude, in part, explains my interest in politics. I have always been keen to see life through the eyes of others. I've had the good fortune to travel extensively, in Australia and overseas, and I've always grabbed every chance to visit people in their homes and to understand their customs and priorities. Five years of suburban life in Reservoir opened my eyes to a whole new set of experiences.

St Coleman's in North Fitzroy was where I continued secondary school. There were fifty boys and a single teacher, a septuagenarian Christian Brother named Brother Bowler, who ran the one-classroom school above another small boys' school.

We had all won diocesan scholarships in Year 7 to attend the one-year program at St Coleman's. These scholarships were designed by the Catholic Church to maximise the opportunity for young Catholic students to win government scholarships in Year 8, four-year scholarships that significantly helped to pay the fees for the remainder of secondary school. In addition to St Coleman's, there was a small college for girls set up for the same purpose.

This was my toughest year at school. Brother Bowler had a nice side to him; it's just that it wasn't apparent all that often, as his mission in life was to ensure that every one of his boys got a government scholarship one way or another. He took his mission seriously.

Classes started just after 8 a.m. and finished at 3.45 p.m. The school consisted of one large classroom, an eating room and an outdoor area the size of a basketball court, with a 2-metre gap around the building and a high brick wall. After we'd eaten our lunch, we were usually given a fifteen-minute break to play. An afternoon break seemed to be optional on most days, depending on the mood of Brother Bowler. It was a grinding experience, and the intensity of the study and the commitment of homework meant that as a class we closely bonded through the shared experience.

This was the first time that I can recall having a problem in the mornings. I would go to bed often close to midnight, very satisfied with the reams of homework I had finished, but when my mother woke me at 6.30 a.m. the next morning, I'd be in a totally different frame of mind. I'd feel nervous and lacking in confidence. I'd be anxious about the quality of my homework, and I didn't want to speak to anyone.

On the three-block walk to the Ruthven railway station I would look at the old, retired men wandering to their front gates to pick up their morning papers and wish that I was one of them, that I'd already been through life's tribulations. I would be very down. Yet half an hour later, by the time I'd caught the train, gone a few stations and met a friend or two and the girls from Santa Maria College, I would find my mood improving.

Invariably, by the time I got to school I was in a totally different frame of mind. I was talkative, confident, optimistic and ready for the day. For many decades I put this morning feeling down to the fact that I just wasn't a morning person, assuming that all those people who said they were not morning people experienced what I experienced.

Brother Bowler tended to have a fit once or twice a week. Drinking water stopped the attack, and a young fellow nearest the science tap on the front multipurpose desk was nominated to quickly fill a glass with water and put it in the hands of the fitting Brother Bowler whenever needed. For the whole of that year, on every occasion, the boy would panic and turn the science tap too strongly, making the water hit the bottom of the glass with great force, and invariably hitting everyone in the first two or three rows. The humour of the situation was lost on many of us after a while because our written work would be wet, the ink would run, and our efforts would be rendered useless.

Halfway through the year, Brother Bowler's superiors decided that he needed a break during the day, so a young brother came to teach us while Brother Bowler was reportedly having a rest out in the meals area after lunch. But Brother Bowler used that hour and a half to comprehensively examine all of our homework books, and we dreaded his reappearance. He invariably returned in a foul mood, and we waited anxiously to see which boy's homework book would be thrown with great accuracy and venom at his chest. Brother Bowler would rant and rave and yell for some considerable time, and meter out punishment, often until it would bring on a fit. After yet another water-drenching episode, calm would be restored. We all won government scholarships and put the year down to a character building experience.

Notwithstanding my great sense of loss, I think the shift from the farm to the suburbs was hardest, by far, on my father. Dad loved the land, the way of life, the independence. It was his sense of identity, an intangible necessity that is important to each and every one of us. But at nearly forty years of age, he found himself in the suburbs and looking for a new career with a large family to support and educate. Neither of my parents ever shirked or complained about their lot.

After trying one or two jobs, my father Frank took a job at WR Grace, a plastics factory in Faulkner. For the next thirteen years, he worked 60-hour weeks, from 7 a.m. to 7 p.m. one week, changing to 7 p.m. to 7 a.m. the next week.

This endless weekly change from day shift to night shift was a gruelling routine, which no doubt played havoc with his body clock.

My mother Marie is a strong woman and a saint. When we were kids, she was always positive (except the odd occasion when she brought out the jam stick!), selfless and generous, and looked for the best in others. She always looked young for her years, and is still the same at eighty-three. Mum would have given Peter Costello a run for his money as a standout Federal Treasurer. She seemed to be endlessly moving money around between all of my brothers and sisters—borrowing savings or pocket money from one of us to pay for school excursions, or some such expense. And she did repay us (mostly). With this came a constant supply of roasts, apple pie and scones, and she still makes a mean sponge. Then at fifty, when education expenses were hitting a peak, she got a job at the St Vincent de Paul stores in Fitzroy and Collingwood and worked there for nearly a decade.

The values, strong faith, sense of humour and commonsense of my parents, now eighty-eight and eighty-three, continues to inspire.

For two Christmas vacations after I'd left school, I joined my father working at the plastics factory, assisting on the extruder floor where he was the foreman. I discovered the great (social) inconvenience of 12-hour night shifts one week and 12-hour day shifts the next.

The one thing I never got used to was the static electricity that was generated by these 10-metre extruder towers. If you had any part of your body protruding, such as fingers or an elbow, the result would be an arc of electricity jumping sometimes up to 3 metres. While the experienced men on the floor seemed to be able to approach the extruder and exchange rolls of plastic or do other maintenance without finding themselves under attack from arcs of static electricity, I never got the knack of avoiding it, and invariably went home twelve hours later with my nervous system well and truly sharpened.

I also had a gig after the factory shift, singing and playing the guitar in a bar called The Branding Iron in Little Bourke Street in the city. I had always sung, initially with a youth group in Reservoir. I couldn't read music, but I had had a few lessons on the guitar and enjoyed the combination of the singing and the playing. It was the time of 'Solitary Man', 'House of the Rising Sun' and lots of Simon and Garfunkel. I also sang at weddings all over the northern suburbs. They always paid well.

When we lived on the farm I had my first experience with politics. My parents were active in the Democratic Labor Party (DLP), which had broken away from the Australian Labor Party in the 1950s over the issue of communism. There was a very strong Catholic component within the DLP because of the strident anti-communist position of the Catholic Church. I can remember my parents discussing the prospects of DLP candidates and the issues of the day. My parents' proudest political moment came during the 1961 federal election, which Robert Menzies won by one seat on the preferences from ninety-three votes for the Communist Party in James Killen's Queensland seat of Moreton. At that election, the Epping booth got the highest DLP vote of any polling booth— 26 per cent. The branch got a letter of congratulations from DLP headquarters, and thirty local DLP supporters later celebrated one night at our farm until 2 a.m., joined by the Victorian DLP Senator, Jack Little, and his wife.

In Year 10, during what turned out to be Robert Menzies' last election and last victory, the 1966 federal election, I asked my father if I could help hand out how-to-vote cards at the Duffy Street Primary School. Interestingly, the local federal Labor member was Dr Harry Jenkins, the father of the current speaker of the House, Harry Jenkins. When the speaker has ruled against me during Question Time or ordered me out of the Chamber, I have suggested to him that it was just payback for handing out how-to-vote cards in 1966 that preferenced against his father.

I went to the Christian Brothers' Parade College in East Melbourne for the final four years of school. My brother Christopher and I travelled each day to Jolimont station near the Melbourne Cricket Ground and walked through the Fitzroy Gardens to school. I enjoyed those years. I worked hard, but they were nothing like the onerous St Coleman's year, even the much-feared Year 12.

Despite already having experienced Australia's ethnic mix through most of my earlier years, Parade College was my first exposure to the different socioeconomic mix in our community.

The shorter school day and easier homework demands meant I had time to develop other interests. I learnt the guitar, joined the East Reservoir tennis team with Christopher, Janet and Beth, and played in the Saturday competitions. And I had a very active social life.

I joined the school cadets in Year 10, but left after eighteen months. The experience left a strong impression on me. I found a lot of the marching up and down and being barked at somewhat futile. I also thought it was an injustice that the students who ended up as the cadet under officers (or CUOs), or as the other officiating officers, were the ones who didn't need to spend their holidays working to supplement the family income. I resented being ordered around by students who only held those positions because they were free to attend the officer courses, not because they had been appointed on merit. Many would yell and scream at you, warming to their sense of authority and self-importance; these were people that I didn't necessarily respect as leaders.

Such was my first encounter with the current head of the Department of the Prime Minister and Cabinet, Terry Moran, a person whose company I have come to enjoy and whom I strongly respect. I remember the Moran brothers well: top-shelf students, standing with straight backs in commanding positions because they attended every promotional course. Meanwhile I was taking orders and working on farms and in factories every holiday.

Every time I have had some such experience, where I have felt I was being denied opportunities solely because of my financial circumstance, or I was being pigeonholed because I came from a dairy farm or didn't attend a tier-one private school, I have got my back up and hardened my resolve to succeed at the highest levels. It has been a great source of inspiration. I strongly feel that you shouldn't be judged on where you come from, but rather on what you can contribute and how you conduct yourself.

The final straw with the cadets came after a bivouac at the army camp Pukapunyal. We camped in great tents and spent the days on various training exercises, including the popular task of firing live rounds at the shooting range.

The second-last evening saw us positioned within a 400- to 600-metre radius of our camp site—half of us attacking, with the others defending. However, our tent sergeant decided that we would do something different, waiting until midnight (hours after the planned attacks) so we could make a surprise attack on another group camped on a knoll away from the formal camp site. Unfortunately our fearless leader miscalculated and we crawled and scrambled surreptitiously past the intended destination and on into the night until we were totally lost. We marched through the night and finally mutinied at 5 a.m. It was freezing cold, so we lit a fire and told our sergeant what he could do with his instructions.

After two hours' rest we set off again and found our way back to base camp at about 10.30 a.m. Search parties had been looking for us since dawn. We had walked an estimated 34 kilometres since we'd set off for a 400-metre surprise attack.

The exercise confirmed in my mind that all of those in authority in the cadets were idiots, which they weren't, but it fuelled my sense of resentment towards them. Three weeks later I got my parents to write a note saying I was not available to give the required attention to the cadets, and I took my leave.

In the end, it wasn't the whole enterprise that I abhorred; it was the attitude of a significant number of these fellow students with officer stripes on their arms. They didn't treat the rest of us with respect; they lorded it over us, even though they were in these positions of authority because of circumstance, not necessarily because of merit. Good luck to them, but they should not have treated me and others as lesser beings.

I believe good leaders don't strengthen their position by putting down the people they're leading. Good leaders have a sense of self-belief and confidence, and they also respect the roles of all those people who work for them. I thought so then and I believe it even more today.

Maureen says I have a chip on my shoulder, and it is probably true that I have always felt driven to prove that no one from a working-class background should be denied opportunities if they merit them. It clearly fits with the Liberal philosophy: if you are given opportunities and you don't make the most of them, that's your choice; you won't be as well off as someone who is given opportunities and takes them. And not everyone deserves to be equal.

Making the most of your opportunities doesn't always entail financial gain. There are many ways we can enrich ourselves, but I think we all have a responsibility to identify our skills and work hard to develop them, and then there shouldn't be too many barriers to achieving that aim.

So I left the cadets and gained more from my holiday work than just the much-needed (and appreciated) financial independence. Christopher and I carted hay, about ten thousand bales, over the Christmas break for a friend, Arthur Christian, who lived at Doreen, just northeast of Melbourne. We milked cows, helped with fencing, went to cattle sales with him and got a very good introduction to commercial life. The money gave us some freedom.

Arthur had taken over his family property aged sixteen when his father died, and he ran the 100 acres with his mother and seven brothers and sisters. By the time we were helping Arthur, he was in his mid-thirties and he had helped brothers on to other properties while expanding the original farm to several hundred acres. He tutored us in business negotiations and life.

He is an extremely astute businessman and has spent the last forty years progressively subdividing, adding more land and subdividing again. He taught me much about the psychology of business, especially in relation to buying and selling, the need for patience and the fact that a deal is never done until the cheque is in your hand or, more to the point, until it has been cleared by the bank. I've been lucky to have a few great mentors, and Arthur was the first.

At that time, he was 6 or 7 kilometres from the fringe of the suburbs, and he anticipated the need for more homes in the future, so he would buy pieces of land suitable for subdivision. He showed enormous patience and astuteness, and he enjoyed doing a deal. Certain deals took years.

Some early mornings at Arthur's dairy farm, I would be bringing the cows into the yard in the dark and would find myself very apprehensive about milking, even though I'd milked cows for years. I used to be annoyed by the fact that I felt like this, but I couldn't help it, and I didn't really have a strategy to deal with it. I'd just try to shake myself out of it and tell myself I knew cows. I was aware I'd feel differently an hour or so later, by which time I couldn't have been happier.

The sun would be coming up, music would be blaring from the radio, the cows were warm and I was in good company. Before milking was finished, I would feel a great sense of accomplishment and I would be positive and ready for whatever the day threw my way.

Commercial options had rarely been discussed in my family. We had owned the farm in Epping, but with the move to Reservoir, my father became an employee. Our parents had a great desire to see us complete education and have good, secure jobs. They wanted to give us opportunities, and with nine children the only way they saw for us to make the most of life was through education. That was a key theme that ran through all of our childhoods. But I really warmed to commercial ideas. I think buying and selling is in my blood on my mother's side. I found it stimulating, but it didn't shake my resolve to pursue educational goals. I think I really wanted to be a farmer, but I could see I would never have the money to do that unless I was rewarded handsomely in some other endeavour. I thought if I could study agricultural science, I could satisfy my connection to farming and the land, and then maybe one day be in a position to buy a property. Arthur laid the groundwork of interest and knowledge about rural property deals.

I went to Dookie Agricultural College to study for a three-year Diploma of Agricultural Science. Fortuitously, at Dookie I was introduced to the study of economics by one of the best lecturers I encountered in eight years of tertiary study. This discipline opened the door to a whole new set of possibilities.

7

DOOKIE

I worked hard in Year 12. I worked my tail off but didn't get the marks to win a scholarship to university. It was a big let-down, but I had also applied for a cadetship linked to the Diploma of Agricultural Science at Dookie Agricultural College, a 6000-acre property that was 34 kilometres from Shepparton in north-east Victoria.

The cadetship indentured you to the Department of Agriculture for five years after graduation, but it meant a guaranteed job. The diploma was a three-year course with a strong scientific component. At Dookie you lived on campus with 120 other young men (at the time they didn't have women students, which we all thought was a great shame). The beauty of the cadetship was that it paid for everything—living expenses and tuition fees—and on top of that I got a $2.50 a week living allowance! I thought I was made.

They were a great three years of my life. It was 1969. I drove up with my parents and a couple of my siblings, and I couldn't understand why my mother was crying when she left. For me it was a moment of great joy and freedom, even though I loved my family. It's a time of life when you can be pretty self-centred. I could go two months without ringing home and then wonder why mum sounded a bit thin-lipped when I finally got around to ringing.

Life was classes, practical work, football and parties. I worked as a waiter at the Goulburn Valley Cabaret on Friday, Saturday and Sunday nights for the majority of the three years. Most of us worked reasonably hard, but we played hard too, and it was a great, formative period of my life.

Johnny O'Keefe, the rock'n'roll legend of the 1960s, played one weekend at the Goulburn Valley Cabaret. I was asked to take a bottle of Johnny Walker Scotch to his room before his performance and then had to pick up the empty bottle at the end of the night. He played for three nights that weekend, and every night it was the same routine. It was an eye-opener for me, a young bloke who had not been aware of alcohol abuse.

The college food was institutional food, but there was plenty of it. If the main course was hard to stomach, we would always fill up on bread and jam. On the odd occasion when there was a tasty main meal or dessert, there would be a race to finish in order to get seconds. Coming from a family of nine children, I was well practised in eating a meal quickly in order to score some of what was left over. This experience stood me in good stead in the college dining room.

Very occasionally, maggots would be discovered in the meat. The meat was butchered at the college and was usually fresh, though the chefs could find many ways to disguise the freshness! An orderly lunch or dinner would be disturbed by the sudden cry of 'maggot alert'. Then all hell would be break loose, with cutlery banging on plates and the cry being echoed from every table.

It was around this time that I also developed severe migraines. I would have one or two a year, usually when we were on holiday. They would last seven or eight hours, and were often only stopped with a morphine injection. (Unfortunately, our son Joe inherited this gene.)

I was elected to the Student Representative Council as the vice president in third year. It wasn't like the SRCs in universities; it was mostly concerned with the amenities and day-to-day running of the college. It wasn't a vehicle for political expression, but instinctively I was interested in that sort of role, so it was probably my first flirtation with politics and leadership positions.

They were three years of minimal pressure, but nevertheless I still found the mornings, or the first two or three hours of the day, quite difficult. I wouldn't want to get up, and I wasn't sociable or confident. But in a place like that, with fellows in their latter teenage years, those traits hardly stood out.

I made lifelong friends at Dookie: 'George' Byrne, Daryl Reid, 'Blue' Lambden, 'Harold' Hooke, Ian Hollick, Mick Keys, 'Fish' Whiting and many more. I learnt to be independent yet part of a group, and I got a very solid education both on and off the campus, especially the idea of not taking myself too seriously—any self-importance would get knocked out of fellows remorselessly by the other 119 students. It was a remarkable environment in that regard, not unlike the army I suspect. And we survived a week of bastardisation at the start of our course. It certainly meant we bonded quickly.

I learnt loyalty and the responsibilities of true friendship. I attended the occasional postgraduate class in drinking, often held in an idyllic learning spot down by the Caniambo River, accompanied by a barrel or two. I could never master the volume associated with beer, so I began a lifetime relationship with whisky.

Playing football for Dookie College hardened many naive young men, including myself, fairly quickly. All the other sides were pre-dominately comprised of mature, hard men, many from the land, with quite a few well into their thirties. Dookie College had never won a premiership, and the other teams went out of their way to intimidate and provoke the young college players, almost all of whom were between seventeen and twenty years of age. It was not unusual to go to shake your opponent's hand at the start, only to be greeted with the suggestion that, 'If you get a fucking kick, you won't leave the ground conscious'. It was a time-honoured and apparently successful tactic.

I was fortunate to attend for three years of the college's golden era of football. We had an abundance of highly talented footballers, and many had a good height and build. We held our own in many of the fights and often came out on top.

We were in the final four each year and won the premiership in both first and second grades in my second year. It was an unforgettable feeling that night, the first time I had experienced premiership success. I was an average player and struggled to get a regular game in the firsts but felt well pleased to captain the seconds to a preliminary final in my third year.

We would visit the nurses' home at Bendigo, a two-hour drive away, and return, not having slept, to play football for the college in the Katamatite League. Some of us played our best football on those occasions. Our relationships with females were shaped away from the critical eyes of our parents, but under extreme scrutiny from each other. I'm not sure which was preferable.

In my second year at Dookie, my brother Christopher and I combined our savings and bought a car—a 1951 four-cylinder, side-valve Hillman sedan—for the princely sum of $120. It turned out the car was worth what we paid for it. Christopher didn't get much opportunity to use it. I proudly drove it up the Hume Highway to Dookie College, discovering it had a maximum speed of about 90 kilometres per hour. It was the last time I made the trip without a breakdown. I drove the car the 32 kilometres into Shepparton for my waiter's job many weekends. Two months after bringing the car up to Dookie, I drove back to Melbourne for a party one weekend. On the return trip on the Sunday night, the car broke down on the Hume Highway between Euroa and the turn-off to Dookie College at Violet Town. Geoff Byrne, one of my best friends, was with me. Despite our best efforts, we couldn't breathe life into the vehicle, so we waited patiently on the side of the highway, hoping other returning college students would spot us.

After two hours, another close friend, Robert Hooke, recognised the car (I have never seen another 1951 Hillman on Australian roads) and stopped to help. We decided Robert could tow us the 50 or 60 kilometres back to the college. The only trouble was we didn't have a tow rope between us. So being enterprising young men from the land, we did the next best thing: we got a pair of wire cutters and took an appropriate length of fencing wire from the top strand of some farmer's fence next to the highway. We arrived at the college safely at 2.30 a.m., though my eyes were on stalks after concentrating so hard for an hour and a half of towing.

The Hillman's motor blew up early in third year. I spent most of the year replacing the motor with another that I had picked up at the Shepparton wreckers for $20. I proudly drove the car home at the end of the year, only to blow a hole in the head on its first outing back in Melbourne … ten minutes after picking up someone I was very keen to impress on our first date. The car went to the wreckers the next day, and the girl declined a second date.

The economics courses of senior lecturer Gary Randall introduced me to a whole new discipline. I warmed to it from the very first class. Gary was a self-effacing fellow with a great sense of humour and a passion for teaching economics. Gary had a bad stutter, and the best way he could avoid it was by inserting the words 'you know' in the middle of sentences, or even in the middle of words. Students would identify his lectures as the 'pro-you-know-duction' lectures.

Economics is simply about finding the best way to allocate, or use, scarce resources. It mirrors much of life. Who gets the last lamb chop? Do we spend our $2000 of scarce savings taking a holiday or building a deck on the back of the house? In this sense, economics is at the heart of politics. Politics is about doing your best to reconcile tens or hundreds or thousands of competing interests. Yet there are invariably too few positions, services or financial resources to fully satisfy the interests of everybody—far from it. Hard choices have to be made. A background in economics helps you make those choices. And so, economics ended up shaping a big part of my life.

Dookie made me think in a much broader sense about my career. It opened my eyes to other opportunities and it gave me three years of experience and enjoyment of regional Australia. It was a diploma course that, in many subjects, took us close to the standard taught in degree courses. This caused great frustration for many in subsequent jobs, where the most challenging work went to those with a degree while those with a diploma played a supporting role.

As a consequence, many enrolled in further degree courses or headed off to do things totally unrelated to agriculture. Some did agricultural science, others did veterinary science or valuing, but I was keen to keep studying economics.

I was locked into working for five years with the Department of Agriculture but looked for a city-based job so I could undertake further studies at night. I had my sights set on becoming an agricultural economist. I took a position as an animal health officer and enrolled in a Bachelor of Economics at Latrobe University. My world was about to change considerably.

8

INHALING WITHOUT SMOKING

As an animal health officer, I had to identify and seek to control any notifiable diseases such as lumpy jaw in cattle, footrot in sheep, tuberculosis, the dreaded foot-and-mouth disease, pullorum disease in fertile hens, brucellosis and other such ailments.

I was responsible for the Yarra Valley district, the northern areas up to Whittlesea, down to Geelong and across to Pakenham. The area ringed the city of Melbourne. I inspected piggeries to see if the owners were boiling the swill before they fed it to the pigs; blood-tested thousands of birds, which was mind-bending stuff; and tested and vaccinated cattle for tuberculosis and brucellosis.

I travelled endlessly, doing postmortems in paddocks, visiting livestock sales, slaughtering diseased animals at the Melbourne abattoir and retrieving organs for pathology. It was a fascinating job, and I learnt much while enjoying the contact with farmers and livestock.

I lived at home for a little while, but after three years of living independently at Dookie I found it hard to fit back in. So I moved into a house in North Fitzroy with a couple of guys I knew from university, with my office just up the road in Treasury Place.

I was able to structure my university course so that I was doing two-thirds of a full load each year, with all of my classes in the evenings. I studied a lot in the library before and after lectures, so I was putting considerable effort into the subjects, but I was always getting Cs and Ds.

In my third year at Latrobe I enrolled in second-year micro-economics, taught by Dr Bharat Hazari, a Harvard graduate. In his mid-semester exam, he set questions like, 'John Dodson owns a milk bar and he's introduced the sale of fruit and vegetables in the shop. It's early in the project but this additional stock is starting to sell well. Discuss'. I was completely thrown. I couldn't see what he was getting at. Nearly everyone failed (myself included, which I didn't like), but I noticed a student, Anne Merton, scored an A+.

I knew her from other classes and so asked her how she scored so well. What had the test been all about? She explained that she had spent time talking to Dr Hazari to find out what he was looking for in the upcoming exam. This was the first lesson I learnt from Anne, which I never forgot: make a point of getting to know what a lecturer is looking for in his or her exam questions. This practice secured me many good marks across all subjects in subsequent years.

Dr Hazari's view was that economics is a very inexact science, that this is not a perfect world, and that with economics you have to assume lots of things about how people will react, how the wholesale price will go up or down, how trends will change. He was saying that there aren't a whole lot of lines on paper; that nothing is a given. The world is uncertain, and an economist has to deal with uncertainties. Sensitivity analyses are important. Assumptions are important.

Dr Hazari was expecting us to identify for ourselves the possible and likely circumstances and assumptions of the milk-bar owner, and to show that by varying these factors you might arrive at different outcomes. We needed to see what was important in different scenarios and what was not; to see what held true no matter what.

It was a light-bulb moment. And it led to the second lesson: the power of critical thinking; of thinking for yourself. It really was the first time I found myself critically assessing issues, challenging conventional wisdom and formulating my own conclusions. It liberated my approach, and I matured enormously as a student and as an individual.

I had long confused uncritical thinking with respect for authority. All through my childhood and teenage years, we were taught to respect authority. For the nuns, the priests, the brothers and many other authority figures, the world was very black and white. We were conditioned to accept their word as gospel.

For me this was exacerbated by a focus on maths and the sciences. These courses and the related books and references were given the status of set truths. But even in the statistics course I was taking, I discovered that the best mathematical brains in the world were all arguing with one another. It was tremendously liberating: to see that a well-researched, considered and argued opinion of my own could be as valid as anyone else's, even those at the forefront of their discipline.

I got an A+ for the final microeconomics test. So profound were these two lessons that I never got anything less than an A for any subject for the rest of my university career, finishing runner-up for the university economics medal in the Honours year. It was a remarkable turnaround for a longstanding D-, C- and occasionally B-grade student. It says much about teaching method, and more generally about the power of insisting that people take responsibility for their own thinking.

The second-year subject on comparative economic systems, and the lecturer who taught it, Professor Laszlo Csapo, were equally influential. He had moved to Australia after the Hungarian Revolution in 1956. He was passionate about the strengths and weaknesses of different systems of government, and the principles and values that underpinned them.

All of a sudden it gave me a framework in which to position and consider Australia and the world. He was most interested in capitalist versus socialist systems, and I couldn't absorb enough of it. He showed the consistent outcome and consequences of different systems of government—why some countries work better than others.

Professor Csapo taught me that philosophy does matter—it matters very much. It was really my introduction to serious politics. It also made sense on a personal level. I had learnt a strong work ethic and had certainly learnt to take responsibility for myself—in a large family you had to if you wanted things to happen. I had also taken on my parents' attitude to educational opportunities. I did and still believe that you make your own success, that if you have knowledge and some opportunities, then the rest is up to you.

Each individual is best placed to determine what they want to achieve, what they can achieve, what they have a responsibility to achieve, and to pursue it. So the notion that the collective good is maximised by individuals having the freedom to decide what is best for them and their families, and then taking responsibility for those decisions, made a lot more sense to me than the idea that a central group is better placed to make decisions on our behalf. It is true politically, economically and socially. However, it wasn't an application of this thinking that led me to get involved in student politics at Latrobe; I just got angry.

It was the early 1970s, before Gough Whitlam was elected and abolished tertiary fees. I was working full-time and paying university fees as well as union dues. Politically it was a very energetic time on university campuses. The Left was very active, and as a consequence the Right ramped it up as well. Student politics was the breeding ground for people like Michael Kroger, Peter Costello, Tony Abbott and other contemporary players. It's where they cut their political teeth. But I was turning up every day after work in a suit and was just focused on getting through the economics degree. To me the activism just seemed like people amusing themselves (I think differently now). I'd had my fun during my first tertiary course at Dookie College. This was work for me.

Latrobe was a new university—it had only been open five or six years—and there weren't many facilities. That's what I wanted my hard-earned union dues to be spent on—food or sporting services—but it was being sent to so-called freedom fighters or was apparently supporting smoking habits. I thought these 'causes' were a load of nonsense and I was outraged that, at the time, I was funding not only full fees but also their own good times.

The Right was dominated at Latrobe by the children of DLP parents, but Whitlam had driven many of them to the Liberal Party. I knew a lot of them from school. So I stood for the Student Representative Council and the Right put me high on their ticket. But there was a guy I occasionally played squash with who was involved with the Left. I told him I wanted to get elected to the SRC, and he must have presumed I'd be another vote for the Left and he got me high on their ticket. I didn't really know anyone all that well on the Left or the Right, but being on both how-to-vote tickets, I came in second in the ballot without one minute of campaigning.

At the first meeting before anyone pigeonholed or 'claimed' me, I declared my independence and managed to be elected chairman of the welfare committee. I could see that was where a lot of the money was being directed. I think it had also helped fund a lot of marijuana, because half the time you couldn't see across the table there was so much pot being smoked.

People would ask me, 'Do you smoke pot?' and I'd say, 'For hours'. You had no choice. After every meeting I would have a terrible headache because of the passive smoking. But I was able to use some influence so that a majority of the money was spent on facilities, such as simple things like coffee machines. That pleased me.

Despite my political awakening, and my clear identification with Liberal values, I wasn't engaged with others politically. I had moved to the economics branch of the Department of Agriculture, so I was engaged in public policy as a practising economist.

I was still working out my guiding principles, but the fundamental philosophical difference between Labor and Liberal was clear to me: the Labor Party thinks that government knows best, and seeks to make decisions on behalf of individuals, while the Liberal Party gives people choices, along with the responsibility for those choices.

That's the core distinction. Philosophy matters. John Howard made sweeping changes to increase choice in schools, for example, and there was a dramatic growth in independent schools in the western suburbs. It was the same in health: 56 per cent of operations now are in private hospitals, so there is real choice, as there is with superannuation. But the Rudd Labor government's instinct in the face of the GFC was to be the only country in the world to re-regulate the labour market, to re-nationalise telecommunications, to seek to introduce a highly interventionist emissions trading scheme, to seek to remove employee share ownership schemes, to undermine private health insurance, to seek to nationalise 40 per cent of our mining sector and to build a massive $100 billion-plus debt, which will mean higher taxation and fewer choices for taxpayers over the next twenty or more years.

But back at Latrobe in the mid-1970s I had just formed these views, and I had just met Maureen. She was studying for a Bachelor of Arts and a Diploma of Education. She had a teachers studentship with the Department of Education. I met her through my housemate and was smitten from the outset. She came from a sheep and cattle property near Casterton in Victoria's Western District, so she was living in one of the colleges on campus. We were married in 1975, within fifteen months of meeting each other.

It was a busy but very satisfying few years. I was playing football or running the boundary for the Diamond Valley League or training for the Murray canoe marathon. I was given a year's leave from the Department of Agriculture for my Honours year, and I was tutoring at night and working during the holidays. I tutored third-year students in macroeconomics at Latrobe University. Invariably they were mature-age working students, so they were highly motivated and often a lot older than I was. It was a stimulating experience.

That honours year I used the nights to do a lot of my work. Often I would study and perform well until 3 a.m., knowing I could sleep for six and a half hours and get up at 9.30 a.m., but I could never do the reverse and get up early. My mornings hadn't changed.

Harry White was my departmental boss at the time. He had a whole lot of young fellows gathered around him, as economics was a new discipline for many areas of the public service. He took an interest in all of our futures. He still does, aged eighty-eight.

I had been working for him for a couple of years when he pulled me aside one day and said, 'Andrew, you've got the makings of someone who can succeed in economics or whatever you choose to do, but you're always going to be held back because you don't realise that there are "INGs" and "THs" when you pronounce words. You'll be pigeonholed because of that. There will be opportunities that should exist for you that won't exist because people will put you in that working-class, unsophisticated box, and if you want to make the most of the abilities you have been given, you need to do something. Go and get some elocution lessons'.

So I did, for two years. I saw it as an investment in my future, as I did all education. I found a retired English teacher and once a week or once a fortnight I had lessons. She used Shakespeare, and it was my first proper introduction to his work, which was a bonus. I not only discovered 'INGs' and 'THs', but I also now have a real appreciation for language, grammar and the power of words.

I had just assumed that everybody stumbled across mentors throughout their life, or maybe I have been fortunate because I'm naturally curious and a listener. But it's similar to what James Packer said in his eulogy for his father. It had been put to Kerry that he must read a lot because he was so well informed on so many issues. James said Kerry responded, 'Well I don't read much at all, but I do speak to a lot of people who do'. I found that if you could get to people who were really the sharpest in their area, invariably they had distilled the essence of their business or area of expertise down to some very simple principles.

Harry White was telling me how I could avoid the categorisation I had already come up against with the cadet corps at Parade College. We all have different skills, and you have to accept the limitations of your own (sadly I was a long way short of being good enough to play football for Melbourne or make a career of singing), but we all have something to contribute.

I was just about to discover that what I had to offer was leadership and strategic thinking.

9

SEEKING A HIT

I was about twenty-eight and, as you do at that age, thinking the world was passing me by. I have always been in a hurry to get to the next stage, and there weren't any more senior-level opportunities in the economics branch of the Department of Agriculture. A lot of my colleagues had won scholarships for further study or were enrolling in PhDs.

I had enjoyed the challenge of my Honours year. The idea of helping to solve a significant problem motivated me enormously, so I investigated undertaking a PhD in economics at a large overseas university. I applied to Harvard and Minnesota, and as a practising economist with a first-class Honours degree I received positive responses, but I needed to secure a scholarship.

At the same time, the newly formed National Farmers' Federation (NFF) was seeking to appoint their first economist. The NFF was created in 1979 and was an amalgamation of all the former national farmers' bodies. The farm vote was diminishing as a proportion of the population and the farm sector needed to be united to maximise its political clout; it needed one voice nationally.

A lot of my economist mates dismissed the job as pork-barrelling for a poorly resourced organisation, predicting I'd be working with generalists on mundane issues, but for me it was an opportunity to get engaged on the big issues at a national level. I was particularly interested in the macro issues that concerned the NFF: removing tariff and non-tariff trade barriers, deregulating the labour market, more efficient and lower taxation, floating our exchange rate, interest rates and stopping excess regulation, as well as national and international banking matters.

David Trebeck, Deputy Director of the NFF and a highly regarded economist, had previously been head of one of the NFF founding bodies, the former Australian Wool Growers' and Graziers' Council. The chance to work with someone of Trebeck's calibre was not only an attraction but also a precondition to considering the opportunity, if it were offered to me. In fairness to my economist mates, farmers' organisations did generally have a reputation as unprofessional, self-interested lobby groups. I saw the formation of the NFF as an attempt to change all this, but subconsciously I think the greatest attraction was the adrenaline rush the job was going to give me. I was perhaps self-selecting for the sake of my mental health.

Looking back on the decision to study at Harvard or go to the NFF, I think I had known, without admitting it, that long hours working on a project by myself would do nothing to help my morning moods. As an agricultural economist, I had been involved in solo projects that sometimes took a month or two and demanded significant amounts of writing. When I was doing this sort of work, I found it very hard to get motivated, especially in the mornings. My mood and confidence would be affected. But I knew when I was on my feet I felt energised and engaged.

I had learnt this dealing with the tobacco growers in the King Valley/Myrtleford area. Historically, each valley had its own tobacco-growers' organisation. Many of the farmers had emigrated from Italy at the end of the Mussolini period, so they had a certain view of government.

The Minister for Agriculture at the time, Ian Smith, was finding it difficult dealing with multiple organisations. Smith called all of the tobacco growers together and said, 'You've all got organisations with assets. I want to deal with one organisation, not five'. It was one of the smallest industries in the state, but still they had these multiple groups. He wanted a committee of the growers to develop one constitution and create an amalgamated organisation. He offered to supply the committee secretary, and Harry White thought I was the man for the job.

It took about five months. First I formulated a draft constitution, and that set the agenda for the issues they had to resolve. The chairman was a young, up-and-coming leader, and around the table were these hard-bitten old fellows, as tough as old boots. Those meetings taught me a lot about the skill of negotiation. It has stood me in really good stead ever since. I have never since been involved in such ferocious negotiations, even having worked with Kerry Packer.

These guys were all leaders; passionate Italians with strong views and forty or fifty years' experience in a cut-throat business. They would be yelling, swearing and thumping the table, or threatening to leave the negotiations. It often felt as if a brawl was about to break out.

After thirty or forty minutes of this, the vote would be put, someone would have lost, and the chairman would move onto the next item. The same person who had lost the previous issue would invariably be putting his point of view on the next item, again with great passion, but seldom referring to what had just passed. I realised the importance of not being moved by the vehemence or threats of opposing negotiators. Once a decision is taken, most people accept it. After a document was finalised with the committee, it had to be sold to the other tobacco grower members. Evening meetings were organised in cold, draughty halls in the middle of winter. As the mere secretary, I expected that my role in these briefings of tobacco growers would be minimal. I was wrong.

From the very first meeting, I was the centre of proceedings. People saw me as the minister's man. I was pushed to the front of the stage and told to explain the deal. It mainly involved about an hour and a half of me being roundly abused, and me abusing them back. I quickly learnt that if I didn't give as good as I got, they wouldn't respect me. Because I was seen to have authority, they took the opportunity to get everything off their chests. Yet every time we went to have a cup of tea afterwards they were friendly and, to some extent, quite deferential. They had had their say, and again I was the minister's man and the Mussolini experience convinced them that the minister was all powerful.

In many ways, that five-month tobacco-industry experience probably changed the direction of my career. I got a clearer idea of what I was best at. I was motivated, effective and enjoying the responsibility. I was getting rid of the black dog a little earlier in the day. I didn't think about it, but I instinctively knew I performed better and felt better in high-pressure situations; if everything was plain sailing, I wasn't in a good space. I think every career choice I've made has been influenced by my pursuit of situations where there are crises and adrenaline.

So, despite getting into the last six for a possible Harkness Fellowship to Harvard or Minnesota, I decided to join the NFF, and Maureen and I drove up the Hume Highway to our new home, Canberra, on a stinking hot New Year's Day in 1980 with our six-month-old baby, Tom, and our pug, Bruno.

I suspect that I was also influenced by the prevalence of sunshine through Canberra winters. I had always found that Melbourne winters, with the heavy cloud cover, really affected my state of mind compared with the other nine months of the year. Being at 1200 metres, Canberra is very cold in winter, but typically with windless, sunny days. We had a house near the top of a ridge above the fog twenty minutes east of Canberra, with a glass ceiling in the eating area. Most early mornings involved soaking up the sunshine. It was a great help.

Fortunately Maureen is very even-tempered and I don't think we have ever had a blazing argument: sharp words yes, screaming never. If we are annoyed with each other, we tend to keep our distance until the feeling has passed. Early on in the relationship, my morning condition would pass by 8 a.m. I don't think I was ever that grumpy in the mornings (I probably was in later years); I was just quiet.

Maureen would always jump out of bed and be the same bright person when she got up as she was all day, whereas I hated getting up anytime and had a much longer morning routine. I discovered a long, hot shower helped my mood.

Finally, I would appear in the kitchen and grunt a few words: 'Hello' or 'Everything alright?' If Maureen was talking with the kids, I just didn't want to join in. Maureen taught, so she would be getting the kids ready for school and planning her own day. So we did our own things in the morning. I could talk if the kids asked a question, but it was just always an effort.

The Canberra job was everything I had hoped for: submissions to the Campbell Inquiry into the financial system; co-authorship, with David Trebeck, of an economic-policy book, *Farm Focus: The '80s*; and representations to the Fraser government on a raft of issues.

As has often happened during my career, opportunities have popped up at unexpected and inconvenient times. So it was, after ten stimulating months as the economist with NFF, the head of the Cattle Council of Australia, one of the autonomous commodity councils that make up the family of organisations within the NFF, unexpectedly retired.

At twenty-nine years of age, I would normally not have been in the running for such a job. However, the cattle industry at the time was in revolt. Low prices had led to demands for more sophisticated marketing methods based on carcass classification, for the reduction of slaughtering costs through the freeing up of the highly rigid industrial relations stranglehold, for cheaper transport and waterfront charges, for disease eradication and much more.

While working as an economist with the Department of Agriculture, I had been involved with many carcass-classification trials and the setting up of a new age, livestock market-reporting system. My earlier animal health experience also stood me in good stead. I won the job of Executive Director of the Cattle Council.

It wasn't long before I got a major adrenaline rush. Three months into the job and the 'Roo in the Stew' meat-substitution scandal broke. Some clever fellows had been putting a lot of kangaroo meat in with the northern Australian lean beef being traded to the United States for use in hamburgers. There was a Royal Commission, to which I had to present evidence. (It happened to coincide with the arrival of our second child, Joseph.) Many involved in the industry did not want to front the inquiry for fear of retribution, but they were prepared to give the Cattle Council chapter and verse, on the condition of anonymity. I was happy to oblige, and duly publicly reported to the commission twenty or thirty examples of criminal practices within the meat industry. I gained a great insight into corruption in various meat works. It was an eye-opener.

No-one was charged, due to lack of evidence. To be seen to be doing something, the Fraser government doubled the number of meat inspectors, which simply doubled the cost for cattlemen. I thought it was madness and a predictable bureaucratic response. It just meant that the cost of bribing meat inspectors had doubled. No-one got fined, no-one got charged, and no-one got sent to jail, but it was all good experience to be thrown into a bear pit like that because the meat industry can be as tough as any industry in the country.

I had really found my feet in the cattle industry and greatly enjoyed it. I travelled Australia; I was in the outback on big cattle stations and met lots of people. I could be mustering, down on the wharves, in the parliament, at sale yards or abattoirs, dealing with industrial disputes, on cattle studs in Victoria or negotiating with meat-industry executives. It was fantastic work and I felt I was influencing commerce in a significant and constructive way.

But within three years David Trebeck resigned as NFF Deputy Director to establish an economic consultancy. I was asked to move to the NFF as deputy with a view to taking over from the incumbent and first Executive Director, Major General John Whitelaw, a lovely man, who was expected to retire within two years. So I returned to the NFF as Deputy Director at the end of 1983, just after our daughter Pip was born, and became Executive Director in 1985.

The day I took over from John Whitelaw was the day of the great farmers' rally in Canberra, and the first day of the Hawke government's tax summit in the old Parliament House.

There was some irony on the day as I spread my time between mingling and protesting with the 40 000 angry farmers out the front of parliament, many of whom were voicing concern about the abuse of union power, and making our presentations to the tax summit, where we joined forces with the ACTU to successfully oppose Paul Keating's proposed GST.

Of course, farmers and cattlemen get up very early, so being sluggish in the mornings was far from ideal. If I was travelling and the farmers wanted a meeting at the start of the day they would suggest breakfast at 6.45 a.m. They would have been up since 5.30 a.m.

I recall ringing the Cattle Council president at the time, Maurice Binstead, at 6.15 a.m. Maurice was a doyen of the cattle industry and taught me much. He had a property at Roma in central Queensland; he fattened 15 000 head of cattle a year. Maurice's wife Doris said that Maurice had left at 4 a.m. to look at cattle in Cloncurry, south of Mount Isa, and would be back at nightfall the next day. I thought nothing of it.

Maurice had a V8 Fairlane and a driver. He preferred not to fly because driving through many parts of Queensland meant that he would see what the season was like and the condition of the cattle. It meant that if three months later he was buying some of the 15 000 head of cattle he needed each year, he would know how they would look, and what he should offer, from what he had seen three months before.

I was in my Canberra office. I had a large map of Australia on the wall behind me, with all the major cattle stations identified. I started to track the distance between Roma and Cloncurry using my hand width. Then I did the same for the distance between Melbourne and Brisbane. You guessed it: Maurice was travelling about 750 kilometres further in two days between Roma and Cloncurry and back than if he had gone from Brisbane to Melbourne. I was amazed. It tells you much about doing business in regional Australia.

Often there were very early flights as well. If I didn't catch the first flight out at 6.30 a.m. in the Canberra winter, chances were that I could sit there for five or six hours while the fog lifted. I could always force myself to get out of bed; it was just my state of mind that was the problem. I would be compelled to engage with people at the airline desk, and would be trying to read newspapers on the flight to get across the day's issues. Sometimes by the end of the flight I was in reasonable shape.

The job increasingly meant I had to confront this depressive condition in the morning, but at the same time the early-morning demands of the job, including unexpected media commitments, accelerated the lifting of the morning cloud, when I turned back into being an optimistic, decisive, confident and strong-willed person.

The NFF was flying high on many issues—it was extremely stimulating. It was the start of the freeing up of the labour market. Almost since Federation, Australia had had a highly centralised system of industrial relations. It was controlled for nearly eighty-five years by big government, big business and big unions. Small and mid-tier businesses paid what they were told to pay as wages, and individual workers didn't get a look-in either.

I was working with the rural industry's best leader over the last thirty-five years, NFF President Ian McLachlan, as well as our fearless Industrial Director and my great friend Paul Houlihan, Deputy Director Rick Farley and our Public-Affairs Director Jeannie Ferris.

Ian led Australia's farmers through some of the biggest economic and industrial changes encountered for many, many decades. He has an extraordinarily keen mind, great strength of character, a sense of humour and an ability to communicate with people in all walks of life. Ian ended up as Minister for Defence in the Howard Cabinet.

Jeannie became government whip in the Senate, and a highly regarded senator for South Australia, before her premature death from cancer in April 2007. Jeannie was a great friend and confidant of both Maureen and myself. Jeannie always had all the gossip. She had been part of Canberra's petticoat mafia for over thirty years, from the time she joined the press gallery in the mid-1970s. Jeannie is sadly missed by so many.

I met Rick when he was running the Queensland Cattleman's Union, one of the member bodies of both the Cattle Council and the NFF. It was an organisation that liked to stir things up, and Rick was the man for that job. In fact, some years later after joining the NFF as my deputy, we came to refer to Rick as the 'stiletto' man. I could take an innocuous draft media release to Rick and he would invariably think about it for a few minutes, add a short paragraph three or four paragraphs into the statement and say it was ready for release. Sure enough, the next day the story would run prominently on page three or five of the newspapers, instead of page thirty-three, and would be leading with Rick's addition. It's why I offered Rick the job in the first place. As a CEO, you have to know your weaknesses, and Rick complemented my skill set well.

Rick went on to head the NFF after I left, and subsequently also made his mark facilitating land-rights agreements between Aboriginal communities and landowners. Rick had started as a NIDA-trained actor and Nimbin hippie. He went on to journalism and became a Whitlam government staffer before heading up the Cattleman's Union and joining the NFF. An unusual career path indeed! Very sadly, Rick died from a brain aneurysm in May 2006 while still a relatively young man of fifty-three years.

The NFF took on major issues. We supported Jay Pendarvis, the owner of a small buffalo meat works at Mudginberri in the Kakadu National Park, in his dispute with the Australian Meat Industry Employees Union (AMIEU). It was a landmark dispute.

The slaughtering of livestock had long been ruled by an award provision that put a tally limit on how many animals could be slaughtered by each meat worker each day. And wages were similarly set by a higher authority: the all-powerful Industrial Relations Commission.

Jay had reached a different arrangement with his workers. They mutually agreed that they would forget the tally, slaughter as many buffalo a day as they could, and work as many days a week as they chose. In return they would be the highest-paid meat workers in the country by a large margin, they would get back to their families in five months instead of six months, and Jay would save the significant cost of keeping this remote works open an extra month. Everyone was a winner.

When this was found out, the union put in place an illegal secondary boycott, stopping any movement in or out of the buffalo works. Jay took the union to court, with the financial backing of the NFF. We raised a $10 million fighting fund. Two years and twenty-seven (successful) court cases later, the first ever damages ($1.18 million) were awarded against a union, along with all costs, which involved another multi-million-dollar bill. The right of employers to negotiate directly with their employees for mutual advantage was established for the first time in nearly ninety years.

Ian McLachlan and Paul Houlihan were a tower of strength through it all. Paul had joined the NFF in 1981 from the right-wing Federated Clerks Union in Tasmania. He is a master industrial strategist, highly respected, as tough as nails; he can talk under wet cement and loves a great red and a 600-gram rare steak, especially if someone else is paying for it. He fears no-one in the union movement, having been belted up more than once outside ACTU congresses in his early days, and still runs a successful industrial-relations consultancy. Paul can often see a good side to Labor governments because he says Labor governments create a mountain of industrial work. Bob Santamaria had been his greatest mentor.

Around the same time as the Mudginberri dispute, Michael Kroger and Peter Costello were fighting for similar principles in the Dollar Sweets dispute in Victoria. They also won a landmark case. We were all young bucks taking on the world. We'd meet in restaurants and trade war stories.

By 1988 I had spent three years as Executive Director of the NFF. I think in most jobs you've got five to seven years to make your mark and bring your own view to things, then it's time to move on, even if you have done a good job. I was still two years shy of my self-proclaimed minimum period in the CEO position, and Ian McLachlan was also finishing up his maximum four-year term as President. Ideally the NFF would have a measure of continuity at the top, and I had every intention of providing it. Then John Elliott came calling.

10

LIBERAL MAN

John Elliot was the President of the Liberal Party, and Tony Eggleton was the highly respected and longstanding Federal Director and Campaign Director.

John Howard had recently lost the 1987 election, mainly because of the highly disruptive 'Joh for PM' campaign, as well as being outgunned by Labor on the ground in marginal seats. Joh Bjelke-Petersen had been the Country Party Premier of Queensland for seventeen years, and had begun to believe his own rhetoric. Supported by some key figures in Queensland, he started the 'Joh for PM' campaign, seeking to capitalise on policy differences with the then federal Liberal–Country Party Coalition, as Australia moved from being a highly regulated economy. The campaign eventually ran into the sand, but not before causing significant disunity and confusion on the conservative side of politics

John and Tony had conducted a review and wanted to fundamentally change the way that the federal party operated. Instead of our autonomous state divisions being wholly responsible for the on-the-ground campaigns in marginal seats, they wanted a measure of federal coordination and a campaigning presence with the state people in these critical seats.

A number of major industrial disputes, including the Mudginberri and Wide Combs disputes, combined with major economic disputes with the Hawke government, had given me a high profile on national issues. So without my prompting, John and Tony approached me to see if I would move to the Liberal Party as Tony's deputy, with a view to taking over after the 1990 election, subject to performance. There were no guarantees, but I had the inside running for the top job if they liked what I did for the next campaign.

I clearly understood what my early departure, along with the retirement of Ian McLachlan, might mean for the stability and momentum of the National Farmers' Federation. I had had no intention of leaving. But at the NFF we had been through the 1980s prosecuting a lot of policy arguments about introducing flexibility into workplace pay and conditions; freeing up capital, financial and exchange-rate markets; and lowering industry protection. Australia and the rest of the world was changing rapidly. The advent in the 1970s of technology that enabled the movement of capital around the world in real time was making all this change inevitable. The NFF had been in the vanguard of many of these public policy debates. Eighty years of stifling regulation was being challenged. I firmly believed in these policy changes and I was very committed to what we were doing. I hadn't previously considered a party-political campaign role because of my policy background, but I realised I had been campaigning for these policies with the NFF.

I was also influenced by the actions of Michael Kroger and Peter Costello. Michael had put up his hand to take on the presidency of the Victorian division of the Liberal Party and was starting a revolution. Peter was being mooted as a possible candidate at the next federal election. I felt that if I was really committed to these policy changes, I should put my hand up and get closer to the real action.

In this sense it was a golden opportunity, although inconvenient for others. It seems that no new appointment has ever been timely for me or for my colleagues but you have to grab opportunities when they come; they may not come again.

Each year while I had been head of the NFF, I had spent a couple of days in December with Ian McLachlan on his Riverina property. We would spend the time discussing what had and hadn't worked in the previous twelve months, and what we would do in the future. That final year, before we went down to his property, I had told Ian about the job offer from the Liberal Party, and he spent a lot of the time seeking to convince me to stay at the NFF, which was his responsibility. By the end of our two days I was inclined to stay put. Ian can be very persuasive.

But another factor came into play. Ian was an independent director on the Elders board; John Elliott was the Chief Executive Officer of the company. Ian and another independent director had taken an opposing position to John and the rest of the board on a significant governance issue, and the split became public knowledge and messy. Ian and John were like bulls in a paddock. The competitive nature of the two men meant that my next career move got caught in the crossfire. Subsequent discussions with Ian, and comments he made to others, sent me the clear message that I should know my place, and that I was to be a 'McLachlan man' rather than becoming 'one of Elliott's men'.

Bugger that, I thought, I am no-one's man. If I went to the Liberal Party I was not going to become anyone's man there either. I resented the notion. No-one was going to hold me back just because it was convenient for him, and certainly not because he thought I should know my place.

John and I had only ever spoken on the phone. Maureen and I, and our three kids, drove down the narrowly gutted Princess Highway a few days before Christmas 1988, and I met up with John for lunch in his headquarters at the Jam Factory in South Yarra. I was shown into the boardroom and asked to sit at the corner of a magnificent antique board table, surrounded by outstanding Australian originals on the walls.

John entered shortly after, full of his famous bluster and with his booming voice. The silver service arrived, along with a very expensive bottle of French red and two crystal glasses. The domed lid of the silver platter was raised to reveal four beautiful Four'N Twenty pies! It was a feast. During that meeting I got no sense that John was going to use my decision in any gamesmanship with Ian. This was a factor in my final decision. He is an infectious personality in terms of ideas and motivation. He crashed and burned—we all make mistakes. We are still good friends. He is one of life's characters.

So, with some very mixed feelings, I left the NFF and moved to the Liberal Party in early 1988. Ian didn't speak to me for two years, but we got over that and remain firm friends.

I discovered an 'upstairs/downstairs' culture between the parliamentary party and their staff, and between elected members of the executive and the secretariat staff. It didn't apply to me so much because of the authority of the position of federal director, but it was alive and well elsewhere. It is changing, but at a glacial pace.

I could see it was my chance to have a significant influence on party policy and structure. I would be able to influence the issues that I felt strongly about.

In the 1987 election the Liberal Party had been totally outmanoeuvred on the ground in marginal seats. Historically the federal party had always run the advertising campaign and the leader's race, but the 150 electorates were organised by the states, so there could be six or potentially even 150 different messages going out to voters.

The Labor Party had begun to centralise its database based on the electoral roll, and they were streets ahead with a coordinated, targeted message across key marginal seats during the 1987 election. In the Liberal Party there was no coordination: each electorate designed its own material with its own message; it was very fragmented. In response, they asked me, as Tony's deputy, to set up a campaign unit within the federal secretariat to work with the states and coordinate the marginal seats.

The states then took responsibility for the safe and hard-luck seats, as before, but in the ten to twenty marginal seats across the country (which might be only two or three in some states), they worked with the federal secretariat campaign officers to provide a theme and message that was fully consistent with the national advertising and the leader's campaign. It meant that the voters heard one or two consistent propositions during the course of a campaign. There would be many issues, but the themes were uniform—for example, 'the Labor government is out of touch' or 'Labor can't manage money'. So a candidate in an ageing electorate might be campaigning on aged care not being what it should be, and would then assert that it was because 'the Labor government is out of touch'.

Six months after I started, Andrew Peacock took over as Opposition leader after ousting John Howard in a surprise attack. This leadership contest was made more famous by the events of the following week, when the key conspirators went on *Four Corners* to detail how clever they had been in planning and carrying out the execution. It left a lot of bad blood sloshing around the parliamentary party and the general membership.

I didn't have a great relationship with Andrew because we had locked horns over issues I had pursued with the NFF—tax reform, exchange rates, interest rates, industrial relations, all of those macro issues that Bob Hawke and Paul Keating were grappling with. Some of the Opposition were trying to philosophically embrace the freeing up of the economy, but others who had long been committed to such things as the industrial-relations club or tariffs were finding it hard to let go.

The NFF had engaged in plenty of fights, especially with the National Party. We had good relations with John Howard as Treasurer in the Fraser government and as Opposition leader, but not so much with Andrew Peacock, who was more old school. However, I thought it wouldn't matter because my task was to set up the campaign unit, and I was totally consumed by it.

Andrew brought Ian Kortlang (who had run Nick Greiner's campaign) onboard as his chief of staff, a crucial and highly influential job. Ian was a debonair, talented, highly personable ex-Department of Foreign Affairs and Trade lobbyist. I quite liked him, but I have never seen a more effective self-promoter. The Kortlang machine (Ian brought several smart people with him) arrived in Canberra and took over the leader's office. They were good operators, but it got to a point where Ian was getting much better publicity than Andrew. Ian and his entourage were required to move on, and Tony Eggleton asked me to work as Andrew's chief of staff. The election was six or seven months away.

I did so somewhat reluctantly. Charming as he was, Andrew had a bad habit of criticising his staff in front of others. I told him, 'I'm happy to come, but there's one condition: if you disagree with what I've done, under no circumstance do you take me to task in front of other people. I will make mistakes, so it is your prerogative to say so. You can dress me down and do whatever you like, one on one, but if you do it once in front of anybody else, I'm out of here'. We shook on it, and he honoured his commitment.

LIBERAL MAN

It was mid-1989 and there was a mountain of work to be done because of the disruption caused by the change of leader and because of policy needs. Parliament often sat until 11.30 p.m. or midnight, but the leader's vote would be paired so he wouldn't need to be there for a vote, and Andrew left at 9 p.m. every night. It went on like this for some time, but we needed greater involvement from him.

Then, three to four months out from the election, he was like a thoroughbred racehorse heading into the straight. From then on, and throughout the campaign, his application was second to none. He worked hard and he is very bright, though he would occasionally not delve deeply enough into some issues, which cost him during the campaign.

Andrew did work his tail off and we ended up as good friends. We still are. He more or less pulled up stumps after that election and went on to another very distinguished career as Australia's Ambassador to the United States.

You can often tell the quality of a person by his children. As a divorced father of three adult children, Andrew was joined for the thirty-three–day campaign by two of his daughters, Ann and Caroline. They were extremely hard-working and effective, highly supportive of their father and a delight to work with.

The campaign was non-stop adrenaline; there was a crisis a minute. The hours and the atmosphere were extreme, and we were in the centre of it for five weeks on the road. We moved everyday, and there would be an office ready for us in some hotel. I never went with Andrew to events; I was in the makeshift office making and taking endless calls. Trouble is, when you are isolated like that, you don't get a feel for what is going on. You are just in a room with problems. You can get very introspective and are totally reliant on the political assessment coming out of campaign headquarters. I gained a keen understanding about what is meant by being in the campaign 'bubble'. The experience served me very well in understanding what those on the road were going through when later I became Campaign Director, working from campaign headquarters.

I blame this false existence for my worst moment in the 1990 campaign. We were taking off out of Perth at about 4.30 p.m. local time, 7.30 p.m. daylight-saving time on the east coast. We had a converted Air Force Boeing 707 dedicated to the Leader of the Opposition and were allowed to use our recent acquisition, a mobile phone that looked like a brick and was just as heavy. The aircraft was fairly noisy and I rang my family. It was 27 February. I had been speaking to Maureen for a few minutes and every now and then I thought I heard the kids singing out something. Then I caught it. The kids were yelling out, 'It's mum's birthday!!' It was unforgivable, especially given that Maureen had been holding the fort for many weeks by herself, as well as teaching English at Merici, a Catholic girls' college in Canberra. Rest assured, I've never been allowed to forget it.

How did I deal with my depression and the pressures of a campaign? Being in a different bed, in a different state, just about every night got to everyone eventually. I had a lot of responsibility and decisions to make, seemingly at every waking minute of every day. The adrenaline never left my body. It was the best antidote for my morning condition, and the little black dog did not get a chance to hang around very long each morning.

After the loss, John Hewson took over as leader and I helped set up his office until he found a chief of staff. This ascension was seen as a move to the next generation after the contest between John Howard and Andrew Peacock during the 1980s. Tony Eggleton retired after a highly distinguished career, and I took over as Federal Director; I was thirty-eight and had been a member of the party for two and a half years.

My aim was to complete the modernisation of the party's campaign strategy. I needed to set up databases so we could be politically effective and cost effective in the way we communicated with people. I also wanted to help develop a solid policy manifesto, which eventually became known as FightBack!

John Hewson drove the development of FightBack!, which some have suggested ultimately became an 800-page political suicide note. There is no doubt that FightBack! had a lot of political ammunition for our opponents, which contributed to our loss in the 1993 election. It is equally true that once we had knocked these negative elements out of this comprehensive and internally consistent set of policies, then in the hands of a master politician they became a great strength of the victorious 1996 Howard campaign. This body of policy also anchored the success and longevity of the Howard–Costello government, because in the end good politics is rooted in good policy. FightBack! gave the Coalition a decade-long agenda. Although John Hewson may not have achieved electoral success, he left a huge policy legacy, which contributed so much to an extended period of national prosperity during John Howard's prime ministership.

Professionally, those four years with John Hewson were probably my hardest. He can be very charming, amusing and considerate, but much of the time he is quite a difficult person to work with, and he wasn't 'of the party'. In politics, in business and in community organisations, your base is all-important. Rule number one is to protect and respect your base. John didn't have a sense of the significance or role of the many thousands of party members, and he never came to grips with the party organisation that is a critical part of every politician's base and armoury.

He had significant strengths. He looked a million dollars, ran 14 kilometres at 4 a.m., slept for only four hours each night, was an extraordinarily good lecturer and presenter, and was extremely good at taking complex issues and explaining them effectively, and at giving people confidence that he had it all under control. He also had very strong policy strengths.

People were just coming out of a recession; small-business interest rates were at 22 per cent; there were one million people out of work and millions of others who went to bed each night wondering whether their or their partner's job was safe. The community wanted change. They were looking for someone who, unlike Paul Keating, understood the pressures they were under, who knew what he was doing. But they weren't in a mood to take on more risk, or to absorb more pain and uncertainty. They were emotionally fragile.

Our big strategic mistake was born out of inexperience; the inexperience of myself, of John Hewson and to some extent our deputy leader, Peter Reith. Nearly two years out from the 1993 election, the Hawke–Keating government started to put the blowtorch on us to release our alternative policy agenda. After five or six months of sustained public pressure, we felt that for our own credibility we had to release FightBack!. So seventeen months from the election we launched the policy to much fanfare and public acclaim. The comprehensiveness of the plan took peoples' breath away.

Bob Hawke, already under pressure from Paul Keating, who was on the backbench after failing in a leadership challenge, had great difficulty mounting a credible response. For perhaps the first time, Bob looked like a rabbit in the spotlight. By contrast, John Hewson was the new generation with new ideas. A man with a plan. Bob looked tired, clueless and beaten. We jumped a remarkable twenty points ahead in the polls.

We did Paul's job for him. He pounced, and Bob was gone from the prime ministership by early December 1991, still fifteen months from the 1993 election.

Paul is a demolition expert. He shut down the many positives in our package and hammered the negatives remorselessly. John was trying to counter by saying, 'But if you take into account this and that and the other, you'll be better off'. But people got lost. There was no answer to Paul's constant and simple refrain: 'You'll be $30 a week worse off'.

Slowly but surely the polls started to slip. And by August 1992 we were in free fall, our private polling showing that we were nearly ten points behind after being twenty points ahead nine months before. This was against the background of a recession that Paul Keating had labelled 'a recession we had to have'.

Paul kept picking on food and the GST, some of the industrial relations components of FightBack! and a couple of welfare issues. While most of us agreed with the policy sense of including food in the GST, Paul had made a tax on food a huge negative symbol of the whole package. The food issue was killing us at a time when people were under real financial stress.

Something had to be done to stop the bleeding and regain the initiative. But John could not be convinced. In fact, he was not listening. We, however, endured three months of lectures and abuse concerning our lack of personal courage, our lack of integrity, our lack of professionalism and intelligence. He rejected the polling. I even received several calls at around 1 a.m. giving me an enlightened character reference. The espirit de corps in the inner circle took a belting.

Finally, in December, three months before the start of the election, John accepted reality and made a number of changes, including dropping food from the GST. We were back in the race. We presented the changes as an example of a leader prepared to listen, and we saw ourselves get back within reach of the Labor government in the polls. But it had been an emotionally searing time.

During those months I had to be in the best possible form. Every day I knew that waiting for me would be a conference call involving the leader, a couple of his senior colleagues and key staff, with a fifty-fifty chance of being acrimonious. Some or all were just as likely to be cranky and annoyed at what they had read in the newspapers that morning, either wanting it fixed yesterday or looking to scapegoat the person responsible for putting it there in the first place.

I needed to be in the best frame of mind; I needed to try to get the cloud to lift as much as possible before I got to the office. In addition to the long hot showers, sneezing and sunlight, I had also read that if you laughed or smiled, it sent a message to the brain to release endorphins, and that even if your face assumed the characteristics of a smile you would see a release of endorphins. I thought I might be able to trick my muscle memory into thinking I was happy and smiling if I drove to work each day with a ballpoint pen in my mouth to mimic a smile. I don't know what people thought looking in their rear-vision mirror, or driving past the other way, but I did it most working days for six or seven years. I thought of it as my endorphin pen. I don't know if it helped. A bit sad when you think about it.

When I got to the office I would force myself to find someone to engage with me. My preference was Vincent Woolcock. Vince was an institution around the secretariat and is one of life's gentlemen, always with a sunny disposition. I could always have a joke with him, no matter what the time. I would seek out Vince to get me talking and laughing, because I knew when I laughed I started to feel better, and then I would start the conference call.

But the intensity of my morning moods was becoming an issue, even though I was still refusing to admit to myself that I had a deeper problem than just being 'not good in the mornings'. Once I was the Federal Director I would have to listen to the 6 a.m. news to see if there were issues running that needed a response. In politics it is very important not to let negative statements run against you without seeking to rebut them, and to put across your own point of view. If you don't answer the attack in the same media cycle, many people will assume that the allegation is true. If we had a problem, I would contact the appropriate Shadow or the leader's office to make sure we had it covered. Over the summer of 1992–93 we continued to improve, we got back to being competitive, and we had something to sell—John was a man who listened. We started the campaign pretty much level pegging. But our plans to transform the economy frightened people, and Paul was very effective at fostering that concern, so they opted for the devil they knew rather than the devil they didn't.

John's visit to a cake shop and his inability later to explain, during that infamous interview with Mike Willesee, how the GST would affect the price of the cake, given that processed food components would be taxed and fresh food components would not, was one of the defining moments in the campaign—if the architect of the tax couldn't explain it, then it must be a complicated nightmare, as Paul had been asserting.

But another defining moment was an impromptu debate hosted by Ray Martin on *A Current Affair* during the second week. It was arranged at short notice, a live debate about the GST in front of an audience. Paul Keating went feral, he just went off his head, showing great emotion and passion about how bad the GST was for everyone. It looked as though Paul had lost it, whereas John Hewson was calm and controlled. We thought this contrast would work to John's significant advantage. Not so. Paul's rabid performance escalated the GST as an issue of concern in the minds of the public and complemented the brutal anti-GST ads Labor was running.

Then the Canadian Prime Minister resigned unexpectedly, and our media linked his resignation to a supposed public backlash against the earlier introduction of a GST in Canada. This quite false interpretation was created by Richard Krever, a visiting Canadian academic who was at Monash University at the time, and who was featured on the first twelve minutes of the ABC's *AM* program that morning, after having appeared the previous night on *Lateline* to speak on the breaking news. The Canadian Prime Minister had resigned because of a huge community backlash over his handling and signing of a North American Free Trade Agreement between the USA and Mexico, but Richard Krever's spin about the impact of the GST became conventional wisdom, and people thought that Paul's concerns had international endorsement and were therefore legitimate—that he had been right to go off his head. From that point on, for the last three weeks of the campaign, people decided to believe Paul Keating and the Labor ads, which were very effective in convincing Australians that the GST would be a disaster for them and their families.

The more the pressure came on, the more John sought to take charge. He wanted rallies around the country. My state directors counselled against it. It was an enormous amount of work to turn out a crowd of thousands, but John insisted. We needn't have worried about crowd numbers. Labor stacked the meetings with unionists who would start mock brawls between themselves to give the TV channels footage of the supposed national division that people could expect under a John Hewson prime ministership. Eggs were being thrown (John famously caught one!); John lost his voice and looked desperate. The mass rallies looked confrontational and were the wrong approach at a time when people were anxious and wanted to see someone with a calm fireside manner. That manner was what got John the job in the first place.

We lost by 1760 votes across eight seats. It was seen as the unlosable election, which we duly lost. It was my first national campaign as Campaign Director.

Election night was a very difficult night. Ron Walker, our larger-than-life and highly effective Honorary Treasurer, had organised a big black-tie dinner for our corporate supporters at the Intercontinental in Sydney. The Electoral Commission had installed a computer terminal up on the fifteenth floor, and the result was obvious from 6.30 p.m. I had to do live television crosses to the tally room in Canberra, and to the national television audience, from the foyer of the hotel. The first interview was at 7 p.m. It was a disaster.

The visual backdrop was of people totally unrelated to the Liberal Party having a drink before they went out for the night. The late Richard Carlton started the interview something like this: 'I am here with Andrew Robb and there's a room full of Liberal supporters who've all got champagne in hand. The top end of town is really here to celebrate tonight'. It reinforced all the wrong images for the Liberal Party. All Richard was interested in was the atmospherics, how everyone felt and what they were thinking. Nothing about the politics, nothing about what seats we may or may not win and why. It was a total waste of time and I refused to talk to Richard again for the rest of the night.

I decided that if I ran the next campaign, on election night I would be in the tally room with key advisors, doing our job. What you say on election night can be very important in framing your win or loss, and in getting off on the right foot. Three years later during the 1996 election, we were working the tally room.

All the while, up on the first floor of the hotel, 150 guests were looking to celebrate our win. For the next two to three hours Ron Walker was pleading for John Hewson or myself to come down, address the gathering and reassure our supporters that what was unfolding on the big screen in the ballroom was not the prelude to a Coalition loss. Somehow I drew the short straw each time. With each briefing I slowly exhausted all plausible excuses for why we seemed temporarily behind—that votes from yet-to-be-counted outlying booths would favour us in certain key seats, that postal votes always favour the Coalition, that preference flows to us were being underestimated ... By my last visit at 9.15 p.m., a reasonable number of empty seats suggested that quite a few people had already worked out the result for themselves. I'm told that some of them left and headed straight for the Labor celebrations! We have a few 'flexible' supporters.

The night only got worse, and then it was 1.45 a.m. and I was sitting with Jon Gaul, a campaign veteran and great friend, working out what I would say to Laurie Oakes at 9 a.m. It hit me that I had to explain defeat. I felt a great sense of responsibility for the loss. I didn't contemplate resigning because of that obligation. For the same reasons, I encouraged John Hewson to stay. You learn most from a loss. I had learnt enough to last me a lifetime.

Paul Keating is one of the most skilled politicians I've ever witnessed. He was ruthless and took chances, such as during the debate, where he had to almost make a fool of himself to get the issue up. He taught me that you need to be bold at times. Despite the conventional wisdom of his party that they were goners in 1993, Paul never conveyed that, or allowed himself to think that, because of his tremendous self-belief. In the 1993 election, coming out of a recession, the people were anxious. They were attracted to his strength and confidence.

By the time of the 1996 election, that strength of Paul's was perceived as arrogance. He was obsessed with the big picture, which conveyed no empathy with people's circumstances and everyday concerns. We very successfully exploited that sentiment. Since then

I've often looked at people who are displaying great strengths and considered how that trait could manifest itself in a negative way. You've then got something to work with.

Our inexperience meant that John Hewson and I got the timing of FightBack! wrong. If we had held our nerve for twelve months and released it three months before the election, it wouldn't have mattered who our opponent was—Bob Hawke or Paul Keating. We would have blown them out of the water. It was such a complex package, it required considerable time to undermine and destroy it.

The trouble with politics is that people believe the bad news and are very hard to convince with the good news. Paul never talked about the good news. Our positive message was less believable than Paul's negative. Another lesson from that period.

There were a lot of us on the party and parliamentary side who could see that next time—1996—would be our last chance. By then we would have been thirteen years in Opposition, and another loss would have demanded a justifiable clean-out at both a parliamentary and an organisational level. There was no shortage of motivation and resolve.

In some ways I was fortunate to be reappointed. We had lost the unlosable. The Liberal Party president at the time, Tony Staley, is a man of enormous substance and political experience, having served as Minister of Communications in the Fraser Cabinet. Tony was another great mentor for me, and a highly effective president. He had confidence in me, as did Ron Walker. I greatly appreciated that confidence and sought to repay it manyfold. I could see why some might have moved me on, but despite losing, or perhaps because of losing, I ended up with a very large measure of confidence because I felt I really had learnt a great deal, and I understood so much more. Also, I had a resolve not just to win next time, but to bury the Labor mob.

11

THE 'BETRAYAL' ELECTION: 1996

As one of the architects of our loss in 1993, I felt a responsibility to put my head up in the media in the weeks following the election. Being forced to confront what went wrong turned out to be quite cathartic and allowed me to keep running on adrenaline for a little bit longer. Maureen said it delayed my personal reaction to the defeat, and that after the early burst I seemed somewhat depressed for quite some time.

I regained my enthusiasm after being included in a political exchange to Japan, with eight or nine others drawn from the various political parties. The current Victorian premier, Ted Baillieu, was a member of the group, and was a constant source of entertainment with his dry and quick wit. The visit covered Tokyo, Kyoto and Kobe, and was extremely well organised and informative—a ten-day introduction to the Japanese political process and to key political and industry players, as well as discussion of major areas of policy. I made Japanese friendships that continue to this day.

My sense of perspective about the election loss was restored. While we were licking our wounds and regrouping, Labor was celebrating. These celebrations of Labor's win, labelled the 'victory of the true believers' by Paul Keating, concluded with a gala ball in Parliament House. A touch of hubris must have clouded someone's judgement, as the media were allowed to film the champagne flowing and the exuberant Labor politicians dancing the night away.

Given what was to follow in the Budget a few months later, we were able to use that footage, featuring a very smug-looking Gareth Evans, to very telling effect three years later when seeking to ram home how arrogant and out of touch the Keating government had become. What was in store for the electorate in the federal Budget proved to be the political turning point of the next three years, and it occurred just six months after the March 1993 election.

In that year the federal Budget was brought down on 17 August. This time the centrepiece of Labor's Budget was an increase in wholesale taxes of over $10 billion. Given that Paul Keating had convinced the electorate that the world as we knew it would end if the GST were introduced, it seemed the height of hypocrisy to turn around six months later and massively increase indirect taxes.

I asked our Director of Research, Mark Textor, to carry out comprehensive qualitative research on community reaction to the Budget. The findings were toxic for the Keating government. We dubbed it the 'betrayal' research, given the profound sense of betrayal identified in every state. The government never recovered, nor did it regain the trust of the electorate.

I have felt the parallels with the first few months of the Gillard government. Despite Julia Gillard promising in the dying weeks of the 2010 election campaign that 'there will be no carbon tax under a government I lead', post-election she broke the promise in order to secure the necessary support of the Greens and the crossbenchers. Again, the sense of betrayal was palpable.

The flip side of Paul Keating's strength, his arrogance, had prominently entered the political frame in the second half of 1993 and it never left. We had something powerful to work with. However, while Paul Keating was increasingly on the nose in the electorate, our leader, John Hewson, was not faring much better.

John had effectively positioned himself as someone not in the mould of the traditional politician. As such, his decision to recontest the leadership, after he had promised to resign if he lost the election, didn't sit comfortably with many in the electorate. Nor did his ditching of his GST as Coalition policy within twenty-four hours of the election loss. John struggled to recover politically. In time, his colleagues came to the conclusion that he was unlikely to lead us to victory, and a number of members were starting to plan his replacement.

This planning was pre-empted by the leaking of a very private and disparaging piece of market research about John to the 7.30 Report. It was leaked from my offices at the federal secretariat. John was justifiably furious. He called a leadership spill in an attempt to pre-empt a move against him. His tactic nearly succeeded, but the dynamic young duo of Alexander Downer and Peter Costello were elected by a handful of votes as leader and deputy leader, respectively.

Although many, especially John, thought I had been responsible for the leak, it was revealed in a book, *The Victory*, written by Pamela Williams after the subsequent 1996 election, that a trusted media adviser, employed by me on a part-time consulting basis, had decided to take things into his own hands.

The morning of the leadership contest was a tense one for me. I was in my office, located two blocks down the hill from Parliament House, with a view of the parliament building. Ron Walker had joined me. If John had retained the leadership I would have been banished, as he was convinced that I was culpable for the leak.

It seemed to take an interminable time, waiting for the phone call announcing the result. It felt like watching for the 'puff of smoke' from the Vatican when a new Pope is elected. At one stage, Ron suggested that I 'stop all the heavy breathing'. I was betraying my tension, something I had learnt not to do, usually, as Campaign Director.

Sadly, the second experiment with younger, less experienced leaders also failed. Alexander Downer is exceedingly bright, somewhat mercurial in nature, but a very effective politician; he's also a good fellow. Alexander's intellect bred complacency at times, and his wicked sense of humour could fire loose cannons. These traits led to a number of early blunders, by which Paul Keating successfully defined Alexander in a highly damaging way. Our colleagues feared that Paul might call an early election to capitalise on these blunders. I shared this view and had very advanced campaign plans in case of such an eventuality.

At the same time, I conducted some very private research that convinced Tony Staley and I that, in the short term, Alexander was unelectable. It was a very awkward trip to Adelaide to brief Alexander on these findings, but he showed remarkable good grace and realism in the circumstances.

Over the subsequent three months, a smooth transition to John Howard occurred. The strength of our win in 1996 owed much to these selfless actions of Alexander and it was a great pleasure to see his subsequent outstanding success as Australia's Minister for Foreign Affairs.

The re-emergence of John Howard was a fascinating political study. In the previous moves to John Hewson as leader, and then to Alexander Downer, the mood of the parliamentary party had been to go to the next generation after nearly a decade of toing and froing between the old guard of Andrew Peacock and John Howard. In both those contests, there was no real support for staying with, or returning to, the old guard. Yet when Alexander stepped down, despite the very high regard for Peter Costello's skills and potential leadership qualities, the immediate instinct of the Liberal parliamentary party was to go to John Howard, a safe pair of hands.

The smooth transition was preordained to the point that on the Friday, three days before the Tuesday partyroom meeting to elect the leader, Alexander kindly consented to me giving John a detailed strategic briefing on where the campaign preparations were at.

After the change of leader, we still feared that Paul Keating might try to take advantage of our weakened position and go to an early election—he should have, just as Kevin Rudd should have in 2010, two months after Tony Abbott took the leadership from Malcolm Turnbull. As a consequence, we had a full campaign organised twelve months out from the election.

For three hours that Friday, I talked John through all the seats, the proposed strategy, the positioning of ourselves and our opponents, the themes and messages, and how we sought to exploit and expose the weaknesses we planned to attack. As it turned out, the strategy was such a good fit with John that 90 per cent of the final campaign strategy was what we considered that day.

John and I had a rocky start when he took over as leader. He had only been in the job a week when Paul called a by-election for the seat of Canberra, as Ros Kelly (of sport rorts and whiteboard fame) had resigned. The candidate for the Labor Party had taken what many people would see as extreme public positions on certain social issues. We did some standard benchmark market research asking what people thought of the candidates.

To get a handle on community priorities, we asked people what was of most concern: the Labor candidate's views on social and other issues, or Labor's inaction on jobs and high interest rates. We also looked at the strengths and weaknesses of our candidate, local newsagent Brendan Smyth.

Canberra is a small town, and one of the 400 people our market research company rang copied down some of the questions they were asked, including those regarding some of the more extreme positions of the Labor candidate. On the Sunday afternoon, one of the newspapers alerted us to a story they were going to run, saying we had been caught out 'push polling' defamatory propositions about the Labor candidate.

Push polling is when someone rings thousands of people at the end of a campaign under the pretext of market research, and puts a proposition to plant a negative idea about their opponent. It usually involves a twenty-second call, not a ten- to twelve-minute detailed interview of just 400 people out of a possible 85 000 voters, nor would it be carried out at the beginning of a campaign. Nevertheless, this is politics, and facts sometimes get in the way. The Labor Party asserted it was grubby push polling, the ABC jumped all over it and the story got legs.

I viewed it as our usual confidential research that we used to guide our thinking and approach. I had seen the questionnaire and had authorised it. The irony was that our research showed that people couldn't care less about the Labor candidate's views, but they were very angry about Labor's poor management of the economy.

But it became a distracting and significant issue. Parliament was sitting that week and it dominated Question Time. Paul Keating was demanding that I be sacked. A lot of my own parliamentary members were angry about the issue, and I sent a 17-page letter explaining events to take the steam out of it internally.

Each day in Question Time, Paul was lambasting John for being weak and for lacking integrity by not sacking me. It was John's first week in parliament as the new parliamentary leader and here I was, his Campaign Director, cruelling his pitch and dominating events. I think John fully accepted that I had authorised the research in good faith, but nonetheless, it was an unwarranted diversion. On this Friday morning I got two phone calls: one was from a senior Shadow Cabinet member and the other was from another Shadow Cabinet member's chief of staff. Both were friends, and they said, 'Look, the word is around up here at Parliament House that John is going to publicly ask for your resignation today'. I thought he was quite entitled to begin thinking that way, given the circumstances, but he had not raised it with me. I also knew that when John took the leadership he had asked several people, including the party president Tony Staley, whether I was trustworthy because I was friendly with John Elliot and had been Chief of Staff to Andrew Peacock. Again, none of this was raised directly with me, yet my tenure was being reconsidered. Fair enough.

I could understand the problem—my area of responsibility had caused a problem for which I may pay the price—but I didn't feel I'd been negligent and I thought that there should be some discussion with me before I got the chop. So I got my back up and called a press conference for one o'clock, didn't ring John, and walked in with Vince Woolcock—a longstanding and respected employee of the Federal Secretariat—by my side. Vince always had the capacity to make me feel a foot taller. He was telling me where the cameras were and checking there were no exit signs near my head, and we shared a joke.

The room was packed with journalists, all expecting me to announce my resignation. I expressed deep regret for how it had turned out, took full responsibility, but advised that if anyone wanted me to go they would have to sack me—that under no circumstance would I resign.

As is often the case in politics, like a firecracker, the issue shone very brightly and then quickly disappeared; life moved on the next week, and John never mentioned my press conference.

John campaigned very strongly in the by-election, which we went on to win with a massive swing of 16.1 per cent, including swings of up to 22 per cent in some traditionally strong Labor booths. A month or two after the Canberra by-election win, things were going smoothly and I was looking for a break from all the campaign preparations. A three-day weekend policy retreat was occurring in the Gold Coast hinterlands at a lovely resort called Gwinganna Lifestyle Retreat, owned by a prominent publisher. The attendees included fifteen or twenty Chinese officials, together with a similar number of Australians drawn from business, politics and the media.

I was interested to meet one member of the Australian delegation from Queensland, the recently preselected Labor candidate for the seat of Griffith, a former diplomat and former chief of the Queensland Government's Cabinet policy office: a fellow named Kevin Rudd.

I had been involved in the campaign that saw the unexpected demise of the Goss Labor government and had heard of Kevin, though I had no real preconceived views. I found Kevin spoke so quickly that my brain struggled to keep up. He subsequently modified that trait. And I didn't warm to the odd phrase or three of Mandarin being spoken at breakfast, particularly when the Chinese were not present. It was all a bit try-hard. I thoroughly enjoyed the weekend's exchange with the Chinese and other attendees, but I found Kevin to be very pleased with himself, and somewhat aloof.

I returned to my responsibilities and announced to my staff that I was expanding the number of target seats by one—we would appoint a campaign officer to cover the seat of Griffith and would increase that campaign budget by $40 000. I said to my team, 'I don't think Australia deserves Kevin Rudd in the federal parliament'. I felt some quiet satisfaction on election night seeing the seat of Griffith topple to us, with Rudd suffering a 7.4 per cent swing in a seat that had previously had a 5.4 per cent margin in Labor's favour.

I didn't see Kevin Rudd again until a chance airport encounter in Sydney in 2000. By that stage I had been in business for three years, and he had finally won the seat of Griffith at the subsequent federal election at the end of 1998, entering the parliament at the same time as Julia Gillard. Kevin came up to me and said, without so much as a hello, 'I know what you did—you may have cost me the Labor leadership'.

It was a remarkably revealing comment and conversation. I saw the extraordinary level of self-belief, the burning ambition, and the long-term planning, energy and discipline that supported that ambition. I was also introduced to a very thick political hide that has both stood him in good stead and possibly cost him dearly in the years since. At that stage, Kevin had been in the parliament no more than eighteen months, had made no appreciable public impression and was already unpopular with his colleagues. Yet he was admonishing me for hindering his prospects of securing the leadership sometime in the future.

As Opposition Labor leader in the 2007 campaign, and on a roll, Kevin tried to return the compliment by campaigning on three occasions in my electorate during the campaign. He wasted his time.

But that was all ahead of us. Despite our rocky start, I thought John Howard and I had an excellent working relationship, and all our endless interactions were always conducted in a highly professional manner. As well as the outstanding legacy he left as prime minister, he is also a thoroughly decent person. Yet I have kept in the back of my mind something that he subsequently told me. He appointed John Moore to Cabinet, and Wilson Tuckey to the ministry, people who gloated so mightily after their ambush of him to install Andrew Peacock in 1989. By way of explanation he said, 'In this business you have to work with everybody. You can forgive but never forget'.

Although John had established an ascendancy after the Canberra by-election early in 1995, many people assumed that Paul would pull something out of the hat and get Labor back in the race. This expectation grew from the 1993 campaign when, by his own efforts, he won what was seen as the unwinable election for Labor.

This was the backdrop to Paul's speech to the parliament on 7 June 1995. The speech made a substantial and very eloquent case for Australia becoming a republic. Great expectations were built up about the speech. The speech and its presentation were statesmanlike and supported a minimalist model for change in moving to a republic. It was hard not to be impressed on hearing it.

Of course, very few Australians would have seen him give this parliamentary speech. Brief news grabs would have been what most people saw. The speech got saturation coverage over the next few days in the papers, with some of the tabloids running full front-page caricatures of Paul Keating dressed in emperor's clothes. The media and commentators labelled it a stunning political initiative, which would put the anti-republic John Howard very much on the back foot, position him as yesterday's man and start Labor's climb back into election contention.

Our internal market research told another story. Market-research guru Mark Textor had devised a way of tracking the reason why polls moved up and down. He took the known strengths and weaknesses, as perceived by the public, of both leaders and both parties. In the 18-month period before the 1996 election, we asked Australians every weekend, via a telephone sample, which leader or which party was best described by a selection of personal or policy strengths and weaknesses. There were twenty-five of these 'descriptors', as Mark called them, roughly half of them relating to the two leaders, and the other half to the parties. For example, we would ask, 'Who is best described as "arrogant and out of touch"—Paul Keating or John Howard?' Not surprisingly, Paul Keating always polled ahead on that particular question. However, the thing of interest to us was the gap in the percentage of people answering Paul Keating or John Howard to each question—how that gap moved or didn't move, and by how much.

The weekend after Paul's speech, this internal research showed that Labor's vote actually dropped two points. And when we looked at the movement in the 'descriptors', the gap of only one of the twenty-five had changed in any significant way, and that was the question about who is best described as 'arrogant and out of touch'. It was the only 'descriptor' to move, but even more significantly it was by far the biggest movement we'd ever seen in any descriptor, and it was all against Paul.

We knew that, rather than being a masterstroke, Paul's speech was seen as yet another sign that he was consumed with the 'big pic-ture' issues and not people's everyday concerns about jobs, mortgage repayments, and health and education services. We knew it cost Labor votes. Our intelligence suggested that Labor did a major body of research once a month and didn't track each weekend. It appeared that they had not been in the field that weekend, nor was it a week-end that the usual fortnightly public polls had been conducted for various media outlets.

The following Tuesday, French President Jacques Chirac unexpectedly announced the resumption of nuclear tests at Mururoa Atoll in the Pacific Ocean. Australia's Foreign Affairs Minister Gareth Evans responded initially by defending the French, whereas

John Howard roundly criticised them and said they should conduct their tests in their own backyard, not ours.

There was public uproar at Gareth's response. That weekend the public newspaper polls were conducted, and on the following Tuesday, Newspoll showed that Labor's vote had not changed and our vote had jumped. The media's interpretation was that, despite Paul's triumph with his republic speech, that success was more than negated by Gareth's massive bungle.

The Labor Party, or Paul Keating at least, seemed to share this assessment, because Paul continued to make the republic a significant issue all the way to the election, including it in his policy launch ten days before election day. So, armed with our intelligence, we decided not to engage in any way on the republic, but rather we let Paul run hard with it, in the knowledge that each time he opened his mouth on the subject it did him electoral harm.

There was no shortage of adrenaline to spark me up over these weeks. And in a weird sort of way, emerging each day from my poor state of mind gave more meaning, and more urgency, to the rest of the day. I felt empowered, free, unshackled and impatient to make the most of the rest of the day while in this front-foot frame of mind.

In some ways, Labor's misreading of the republic issue had had its genesis three decades before, with Gough Whitlam's ascendancy to the leadership of the Labor Party in February 1967. The Labor Party grew out of the union movement. For many decades they represented overwhelmingly the workers and their families. Gough saw a need to broaden Labor's base if Labor was to survive and succeed long-term. Also, Gough was not 'of Labor', in the sense that he grew up in a middle-class, intellectual, socially progressive environment. Gough wasn't a man familiar with the financial struggles and the social conservatism of the 'workers'. So he set out to broaden Labor's political base by welding the socially progressive middle class onto Labor's traditional working-class base.

Many of the new Labor MP's in the 1970s had not trodden the traditional route from a working-class, socially conservative background to 'shop floor', union representative, assistant secretary or secretary of a union, and then into parliament. Increasingly, the route involved a middle-class, socially progressive background, university, then either straight into a politician's office, the party machine, a law firm concerned with 'rights' issues or a position as a union research officer, assistant secretary or secretary, and then into parliament. All of these jobs are largely campaigning-type roles. The problem for Labor is that the values, priorities and interests of these two categories of Australians are very often diametrically opposed.

By the 1980s, the composition of the Labor Party caucus was well into this transition. However, the workers stuck with Labor because they trusted Bob Hawke to look after their interests. But with Bob ousted in 1991, many Labor voters were ready to consider the conservative side of politics, but FightBack! was a step too far.

By 1996, we had finessed our policies and the people had experienced three more years of Paul Keating, whose 'strength' in the 1993 election had quickly morphed into 'arrogance' and lack of interest in the everyday worries and priorities of working families. And so 'Howard's battlers' were born. A socially conservative son of a local garage owner and war veteran in suburban Sydney was seen to show far more empathy with many in Labor's traditional base than a French clock–loving, 'big-picture' Paul Keating.

This conundrum for Labor has only grown. In 2011, its caucus is comprised largely of political suits. Most of its Cabinet have followed the 'new Labor' path identified earlier, including the current Prime Minister and Deputy Prime Minister. There are many smart and personable people among the Labor members and senators, with presumably noble intent, but their career backgrounds are over-whelmingly highly focused on campaigning and political marketing (aka spin). Their ability to put themselves in the shoes of so many other sections of our community, including their traditional base, has been highly compromised.

Paul Keating did us another favour in the year leading up to the March 1996 election, in his dogged and almost self-indulgent defence of the Labor Member for Fremantle, and former premier of Western Australia, Carmen Lawrence. She faced a WA State Government–initiated royal commission into her actions, when premier, in seeking to sully the reputation of Richard Court, then Opposition leader. It came to be known as the Penny Easton affair, with Carmen famously responding, 'I don't recall' to many questions. For many months in the middle of 1995, every time Paul Keating and Labor looked like getting some political traction, the inquiry would raise its head again, with Paul wading into it, causing yet another damaging political distraction for Labor's campaign. For us, it was the political gift that kept on giving.

But by October, Paul started to apply very effective pressure on us to release policy details. He was looking for a target. Through the year, John Howard had given a series of 'headland' speeches, which sought to clearly identify our priorities and the direction in which a Howard government would take Australia. However, we had withheld much of the specific detail for release closer to the election, to minimise the opportunity for Paul to do what he had done so effectively in the lead up to the 1993 election with Fightback!. Nevertheless, the criticism and demands for release of policy detail by Labor and commentators was becoming relentless. It spooked many of our candidates and poli-ticians, and their campaign teams. By early December, the telephones were running hot, particularly to John Howard, with colleagues sug-gesting he was putting our election prospects at risk.

I knew, and John knew, that if we could hold off releases of major details until the end of the year, then we had enough well-developed policies to allow us to release one a day for three months. This would give us great momentum. I was very much hardened by the experience of the 1993 election, and very strongly argued for sticking to our original plan. John decided to tough it out, even though it caused considerable internal angst. He made the right call.

With the dawn of the new year, we released a policy a day until the election on 13 March 1996. As Labor sought to respond to one policy, we were on to the next. It worked magnificently. We looked energetic, well prepared and forward focused. This strategy anchored a powerful campaign and frustrated Labor.

In the middle of our campaign, we announced that we would establish a $1 billion environmental heritage fund that would be funded by some of the proceeds of our proposed sale of Telstra. The financial commitment took the community's breath away, and it highlighted our credentials as serious environmental managers. The community was comfortable with our proposal to prioritise the environment, and we gained the support of the forestry and farming industries, as well as the Australian branch of the World Wild Fund for Nature. Alec Marr, the then senior Wilderness Society organiser, attended our launch. Paul was not happy.

Our Shadow Environment spokesman and a good friend of mine, Rod Kemp, had very effectively spearheaded this initiative for over twelve months. Given my campaign role, my agricultural background and my contribution to establishing 'Greening Australia' when I ran the NFF, Rod had invited me to be extensively involved. I travelled with the forestry industry and later with the WWF to inspect all the areas of major concern in Tasmanian forestry, and was involved in the myriad negotiations over many months. Establishing the fund, and gaining such widespread support, was a source of considerable pride for us all.

We were also justifiably proud of the way we had communicated effectively and directly with individual voters, particularly in the marginal seats, using the national database and the related software we had built since 1990. The database was based on the electoral roll.

My Deputy Campaign Director, Lynton Crosby, was responsible for running all of our marginal-seat campaigns across Australia. Lynton, a very good friend, succeeded me as federal director in 1997 and went on to direct two very tough but successful campaigns in 1998 and 2001. He is an outstanding professional and now runs, with Mark Textor, his own international firm, which recently directed the highly successful campaign that installed Boris Johnson as London's mayor.

Between the 1993 and 1996 campaigns, we greatly enhanced this database by spending millions of dollars directly contacting and identifying swinging voters, asking them about their concerns, their priorities and their wishes. We asked permission to contact them with information about these concerns as the election grew closer. So, during the campaign, when Lynton and I would be told at 5.15 a.m. that our polling had discovered overnight that 25–39-year-old women had moved against us on health in four seats in southern Queensland, we would respond by communicating directly with those disaffected voters. By 11.30 a.m., a letter would have been dispatched to all those swing voters we had identified in those electorates who were 25–39-year-old women concerned about health. In this way our communications were personally relevant. We saved the millions of dollars it cost over three years to assemble all that information through the substantially smaller specific mailings, and call-centre contact. We saw a dramatic improvement in the effectiveness of our direct communications. The positive response was immediately observable in subsequent nightly polling.

John Howard was in his element during the election: experienced, focused, thorough, in control and enjoying the smell of battle. On the very odd occasion that he tripped up, he had the good grace and common sense in the morning telephone hook-up of the leadership team to say up-front, 'Good morning everybody. I had a problem or two yesterday. We've got a few bad headlines; I apologise'. You could almost hear a collective sigh of people breathing out; Oh good, we can move on. The issue was gone; people could then talk freely about anything.

People now often ask how I could cope in election campaigns with my morning problems. In many ways I looked forward to those hectic, adrenaline-filled weeks. Typically I got to bed between 11 p.m. and 11.30 p.m., and rose each morning at 4.30 a.m. for our daily 5.15 a.m. meeting. The adrenaline never seemed to leave my system. I would be lacking in some confidence when I got up, but by the time I had spent thirty to forty-five minutes assessing the overnight polling and media, and making decisions about the day with my five most senior colleagues, I would be riding high with adrenaline and starting to feel normal. The first three hours of every day was non-stop decision-making, opinion-forming and high-level communications with the parliamentary Leadership group, before heading off with a few colleagues for an 8 a.m. breakfast and more discussion. I have always held up well for the campaigns, except for the last day or two. Invariably I have developed a bad cold at the end of each campaign. I suspect that once my body wasn't feeding off adrenaline, my immune system collapsed.

We worked right through the 1996 election day—doing radio interviews, getting readings from my state directors on the mood at polling booths around the country, getting the exit polls, moving to the national tally room, briefing our panel members involved in the TV coverage, and doing interviews on the floor of the tally room about the most up-to-date results. Finally we had a champagne—we had recorded the biggest Liberal win in history—but in the anteroom, not in front of the cameras. We were conscious about the perception of new government and didn't want to repeat the misjudgement of Labor's 1993 celebrations.

Over the subsequent months in government, my respect for John's capacity to handle mountains of pressure grew. In particular, the first twelve months saw a number of ministers resign because they had breached, usually unwittingly, a code of ministerial conduct introduced by John. Some were close friends of his, and he took it hard. It caused a lot of unease within the team and drew considerable public criticism. Over this period, John's wife Janette was also battling with cancer. It was not a great start.

Some days you could see he was under considerable strain, but he always understood there had to be decisions taken now that were necessary to see things delivered in six, nine or twelve months' time. He understood other people had to keep going on other issues, no matter what crisis he was confronting. John was experienced enough, and had enough character, to be able to compartmentalise things, go and take other important decisions, then come back and join the crisis, but without all the yelling and histrionics of many other leaders.

John's first term was a remarkable term of reform. It included: the toughest Budget in decades because of the $96 billion debt and $10 billion deficit left by Labor; the reform of the waterfront; development and successful presentation of the GST to the people at the subsequent election; strong leadership of Australia through the Asian financial crisis; introduction of gun control; part sale of Telstra; workplace-relations reform; and the national environmental package.

During the campaign, the award-winning *Australian Financial Review* journalist Pamela Williams had asked me to help give her an insight into the 1996 election campaign, which included some exposure not only to the leader and his travelling team, but also to the dynamics of the campaign headquarters (CHQ). Having a journalist visit CHQ was unchartered waters. There was great concern about our 'secrets' getting out. I didn't see any real harm being done, as long as it was managed.

Pamela really had one extensive opportunity to tour our headquarters in a rented space in Exhibition Street in Melbourne's CBD. She observed the tactics team in action fighting political bushfires; the agency people led by Mark Pearson and his creative genius, Ted Horton, turning around TV ads in half a day; thousands of targeted direct-mail letters being written, printed and despatched; the media monitors, the policy wonks, the many people supporting marginal seats with ideas, graphics, defence material, tactical advice and encouragement; the 'top secret' polling office led by Mark Textor; strategy meeting preparations for a press conference; our technical and administrative support staff and our five receptionists. All eighty-four members of our headquarters staff were hand-picked for their political experience.

I met Pamela on a regular basis for an update and a coffee, and approved such meetings with Lynton Crosby, Mark Textor and Jon Gaul, the very experienced head of our tactics team.

Pamela filed some excellent features on the campaigns of both major parties in the aftermath of the election, bringing a unique perspective. Six months later she started work on her book, *The Victory*. By then I was living and working in London for two months, at the invitation of the Conservative Party, to do an independent review of John Major's campaign, five months before the scheduled UK election. I'd said I would do the review of the campaign if I could bring my own researcher and we could do our own research, not relying on the Conservative Party's work. So we appointed a local research moderator to work with Mark Textor, and the three of us set off by train to travel the length and breadth of the UK, sitting in living rooms in a different city each night with local focus groups, trying to assess the political mood and concerns of the average Brit.

During this time, Pamela continued her research about the Keating/ Howard campaign, ringing me two or three times a week for several weeks, asking for endless detail about each day of the Australian campaign, the issues, what happened, how and why. Despite the level of contact, I had no idea that the book tracked the campaign through the eyes of the two campaign directors—myself and Labor's National Secretary, Gary Gray. Alternate chapters revealed how the many issues and events were dealt with by each campaign.

Pamela's anecdotal style of writing gave great life to the ebb and flow of the campaign, to the crisis-a-minute nature of many days, to the tactics and techniques employed by both camps and to the daily tensions, disagreements, little triumphs and routines. It was a good warts-and-all account of how the contest was fought, from an untold perspective.

Some people were annoyed that I had revealed some of our campaign techniques. We were ahead of Labor in some areas, but that is usually only temporary. We both have smart operators; we all watch what each other does, and we both have strong connections to North American and European parties. In the end it is the knowledge of the campaign principles that matter, and your experience. And, as a student of Machiavelli, I'm convinced that the principles haven't changed in 500 years. A searing loss or two won't go amiss either in the learning process. I had no intention of writing a campaign book, and I thought Pamela's book gave me an opportunity to pass on to our younger campaigners some of the things I had picked up along the way, even if it meant sharing it with our opponents.

I also heard that there was considerable resentment within the Howard family that John didn't feature more in the book. I had no way of influencing Pamela's approach and I thought *The Victory* was highly complimentary of John, as it should have been, because he did such an outstanding job. Paul didn't fare so well. Nevertheless, it was suggested I should keep my distance for a while. I have never discussed the book with John, so he might not have cared, but I think it did stick in his craw. Towards the end of his time as prime minister, Maureen and I got back on the invitation list for Christmas drinks at Kirribilli House.

12

LIFE WITH THE PACKERS (AND OTHERS)

I think running two federal campaigns is enough for most people, and I had been Andrew Peacock's Chief of Staff for another. I had already decided a year or two out from the 1996 election that if we won, I would pull up stumps twelve months after the election. At forty-five years of age, I had other things I wanted to do. I also believed that it was time for someone with a different perspective to take over. People start with a lot to offer; they put their stamp and experience on an organisation, and then it's time to move on. I had been in politics for nine years.

I was keen to stand for parliament, but first I wanted to gain more business experience and be better established financially so that if I did enter parliament, I could concentrate fully on the job at hand, and not be worried about our finances.

Our children Tom, Joe and Pip were then seventeen, fifteen and thirteen respectively. They didn't want to leave their schools and friends in Canberra, but the business opportunities for me lay in Sydney. Our kids had not needed to confront such an upheaval before, and while it was tough, we thought it would be good for them. Life is full of change. Despite the early tears and natural apprehensions, it has turned out very well. They have all made lifelong friends at school and during their tertiary education, and are making a good fist of life in Sydney. Maureen and I are very proud of them. Most importantly, we are a very close-knit family, despite Maureen and me leaving them unexpectedly seven years after moving to Sydney, when I stood for preselection in the Melbourne bayside seat of Goldstein.

I had told John Howard and Tony Staley two or three months after the 1996 election that it was likely that I would leave within the year. I had already had some discussions with James Packer, and he and his father Kerry were keen for me to join their company, Publishing and Broadcasting Limited (PBL), initially to assist in negotiating with the federal government in relation to legislation dealing with the introduction of digital television.

I couldn't join the Packers for a few months because of other contentious media legislation already before the parliament. If I had joined PBL in the middle of parliament's consideration of that legislation, there would have been claims of unfair influence. The Bill would have failed, and I would have been the culprit. As it was, that Bill still failed to get passed by the Senate some months later.

So I took up a six-month project with the Commonwealth Bank of Australia (CBA), working with their longstanding and highly respected Chief Executive Officer, David Murray. That time gave me a great insight into banking, and I made many enduring contacts, including Lyndal Fraser, who first recruited me. The six-month bank project involved a highly sensitive commercial issue, which needed a campaign approach if it was to be successfully resolved. I was contracted to help coordinate the campaign.

The project, which must remain confidential, found me working across most sections of the bank and gave me a fascinating introduction to the culture and operations of such a huge organisation. While

I greatly enjoyed the experience, and the project was very successful, I realised such an environment was not for me. With 41 000 staff at the time, I can't recall going to an internal meeting where there weren't seven to ten CBA executives, from a multitude of branches. Big companies, like the public service, are highly bureaucratic. Yet I also found how powerful a juggernaut a large bank is. I would see mistakes made that I thought would have a material impact on the business, yet with over seven million customers, it was like being onboard a giant supertanker that just keeps ploughing on.

My family didn't move to Sydney until the end of 1997, so during my six months with the CBA I returned home to our Wamboin property each weekend. During the week, I stayed at the York apartments, which looked straight down to the city entrance of the Sydney Harbour Bridge, and across the bridge itself. The traffic lights at night were spectacular. The apartment was very comfortable, and I learnt to cook more than bacon and eggs, and vegetable soup.

My morning problem had started to extend beyond 8.30 a.m. some days, and it wasn't helped by my daily ten-block walk to the CBA headquarters from the York apartments. The Sydney skyscrapers mean that there is no direct sunlight in much of the CBD before 9.30 a.m. In winter, the wind-tunnel effect of the buildings made the walk a remarkably cold one. The cold and this lack of sunshine compounded my negative state of mind.

I'd met Kerry and James Packer a few times, but I didn't know them well. I had first been involved with them during the landmark Mudginberri abattoir dispute in the mid-1980s, when I headed the National Farmers' Federation. Kerry had big pastoral and abattoir interests, was supportive of what the NFF was doing, and helped us financially to take on the Australian Meat Industry Employees Union in the landmark dispute. It was at this time that I first met Malcolm Turnbull, who was Kerry's young general counsel. Kerry was a fascinating character. I have always been attracted to people who make things happen.

Compared with the huge hierarchy and bureaucracy of the big banks, it was the complete opposite at the Packers. They always have projects on the go, and issues are constantly emerging, but it is quite informal; there are fewer defined executive positions—I didn't have a title, my business card just said 'executive'—and that is what I liked about the place. No-one seemed too fussed about those sorts of things. The Packer organisations employed tens of thousands of people, yet the structure was very decentralised. Their various business entities were given considerable autonomy and responsibility, with a small corporate headquarters comprising Kerry and James, a group of five or six senior executives, a few analysts, legal people and support staff overseeing the group of companies.

I had always been impressed by the culture of the place. It is true it was blokey, despite the number of strong women working within many of their businesses. You knew where you stood. Good times were had, but business was always the central focus, and if they trusted you, they gave you great loyalty. That was evident as soon as I got there: if you showed loyalty to Kerry, then he returned it in spadefuls, and James was the same. I suspect they are forever looking at the motives of people in terms of their friendships and alliances; no doubt they've been bitten more times than they would care to admit, because people can be very duplicitous. Trust was the most important thing to them, then everyone could be honest with one another, and if a mistake was made, you were told to your face and the air was cleared.

A few months after starting with the Packers I found myself meeting for an hour with Thailand's largest telecommunications owner, Thaksin Shinawatra. Thaksin was visiting Australia wearing his telco hat, but he was also seeking informal political meetings with people of political interest to him. After he met with Kerry, I had a stimulating discussion on political strategy, campaigning and party structure. Thaksin left without alerting me to his political plans.

Two weeks later, in March 1998, my office phone rang and it was Thaksin in Bangkok asking whether I would consider coming to Thailand for two months to advise him on setting up his new nationwide political party, and to train some of his people in campaigning. I went and saw Kerry and his response was, 'What are you waiting for? On your bike'.

I helped Thaksin plan the creation of the political party called Thai Rak Thai (Thai Loves Thai), and then ran a series of campaigning seminars with senior members of the political team that he had already assembled. It was fascinating to immerse myself in the politics of an Asian country, to explore the cultural and historical drivers, to seek to cut through the traditional Asian model of coalitions of influential parliamentarians from different regions and to have input into developing a philosophical base for this nationwide party.

Before arriving at PBL, I had an impression, perhaps born out of Kerry's celebrity status, that a lot of decision-making was made on the run. Yet this was far from the truth. What I found when I was back at PBL was a series of highly professional investment teams, gathering some of the best minds from the investment banks, and from law and accounting firms, without having a big bureaucracy to support. These people were expensive, but they could give the best advice, were extremely well connected, and could be trusted to keep a confidence. And once it was over, it was over. They went back to their firms. With this approach, any opportunities across the PBL/Australian Consolidated Press (ACP) group of companies, and beyond, were very rigorously put under the spotlight. Whatever you were working on, you didn't talk to anyone about it other than those in the group that had been established around the project.

Sometimes there might be up to twelve months of serious work undertaken, and then the investigation might stop overnight.

I was on one project (they all had code names) that concerned a potential hostile takeover of a major Australian brand-name company. It had been worked on secretly for over year. I had set up a war room with eighteen people where we workshopped every eventuality if and when the play was made—what the target company might do, what we might do depending on what they did—covering several possible outcomes. I had set up computers, databases and communications ready to handle a sophisticated takeover bid.

One day the share price of the potential target went up by a dollar and I got a phone call that night. It was off. I was to dismantle everything and head back to my usual office at PBL's Park Street headquarters as soon as I was done. It took a couple of days to wind everything up and close things down, and when I got back to Park Street, I expected to get an explanation, but to this day I don't know the full reason for their decision. At 10.30 a.m., I was called into James' office—the debriefing, I thought—but it was about another, unrelated issue, and he made no mention of the takeover project. I never heard any more about it. Amazing, but it exemplified the way PBL runs: everything is on a need-to-know basis.

Kerry was the dominant figure at the company pretty much until the end of his life, but James had a big influence in the digital area, and Kerry backed him. It is one of the few companies that made serious money ahead of the 'tech wreck'. They publicly floated the company, ninemsn, and realised a huge capital gain.

Clearly Kerry's heart was in television; James' much less so. Kerry loved sitting at home watching television and figuring out what the next trend would be and why people liked certain programs. He had a real common touch. James' passions were more new media, casinos and related tourism businesses.

I learnt much from my involvement with a small number of these investment teams, yet my primary responsibility was to coordinate our negotiations with government over the proposed digital-television legislation. I travelled a lot, especially to Canberra, getting as much intelligence as I could and seeking to influence the government's approach to the legislation. Given the huge expense associated with the transition to digital television, PBL was particularly concerned that additional free-to-air channels not be introduced. I was up against an old friend and colleague, Graham Morris, who was working for the Murdoch camp. Graham had a lot of political experience, including being my deputy in 1992–93, State Director of the Liberal Party in South Australia, and Chief of Staff to Prime Minister John Howard in 1997–98.

Days in Park Street started at 7 a.m. or 8 a.m., and you were expected to hit the ground informed. I had an office on level three without a window, which was not good for me, particularly in the mornings. So I found myself a nearby cafe—Bambini Espresso—in Elizabeth Street, which faced east. In the morning, the sun would be streaming in the window, and I arranged meetings at the cafe from 8.45 a.m. onwards. Sometimes I spent much of the morning in the cafe. In between meetings, I would read the papers there and absorb the sunshine and the stimulation of people around me. It meant that by the time I got to my office I was firing.

If I had an early morning meeting with Kerry, I would have to be on my toes immediately. He was a very challenging man, and he could spot weakness in people. He would often pose questions in such an aggressive manner that people felt obliged to give an answer, even if they really weren't sure. Bad idea. An hour later they would still be wishing they had kept quiet as Kerry taunted them. I was determined that if I didn't know something, I would say, 'I don't know the answer but I will get back to you'. Sometimes he would fire three, four or more questions in a row that I wasn't sure about, and I'd have to answer the same way each time. He would bridle, but he had to accept it. Invariably he'd forget all about it anyway.

One day I was in his office by myself, and we were talking about a running issue in the beef industry. Because of my past work, I knew animal economics as well as my way around an abattoir.

In the middle of the conversation, he said something about the cost and economics of certain abattoir practices, and I said, 'I don't think that's right'. As soon as I said that, I realised I hadn't been involved in the meat industry directly for some years, but it was too late. He had me. He thundered, 'What do you mean?'

I put my case and he put his great big paw of a hand on the phone, lifted it and said, 'Get me whoever', 'whoever' being the managing director of the biggest abattoir in the country, which Kerry part owned with Teys Bros. We sat there while his PA was getting the other person on the phone, and he didn't say much more. I could see his mind thinking he was going to have some fun.

The two-minute wait felt like ten. So the fellow came on the line and they had a bit of a chat about other things just to prolong the agony. Then Kerry started to ask about whatever we had been arguing about. Then he gave a really dismissive grunt, said, 'OK' and slammed down the phone. The gods were on my side that day. 'You're right', he said. He was big enough to admit it, but I never let my guard down again after that. If I wasn't certain, I'd repeat the mantra—'I don't know the answer but I'll get back to you'.

I saw it as his version of fly-fishing, hooking the unsuspecting and exposing their ignorance on some matter or other. He was a fascinating man with his own demons. The only time I felt he was really enjoying himself was when he was in the middle of a deal. That is when I think he was at peace—when something big was happening and he was in the thick of it, negotiating.

There was a great energy about the place. There was a sense that exciting things were happening; everyone was looking for opportunities, and if they didn't work out, they weren't looking to blame people. If you did well, you were rewarded, and things moved on. If you had made a mistake, you got told, and things moved on. If you made a number of mistakes, you were moved on!

There seemed to be quite a strong respect between the Murdoch and Packer camps. They have spent a lot of time scheming against one another over the last fifty years, but there was great mutual respect, and the ability to team up when it was advantageous to both. For someone looking for adrenaline, it was a highly stimulating environment.

After about eighteen months the negotiations over the digital-television legislation were coming to a satisfactory conclusion, from our point of view. I told James I would be grateful if I could get a more hands-on commercial opportunity. Again I was in a hurry to get more experience. He said it was up to me to come up with an idea they could consider investing in. To this end, my political experience in building and enhancing a voter database, and in carrying out sophisticated, targeted direct mail communications, came in handy.

The first thing I observed was that the PBL/ACP group of companies was in possession of an unbelievable amount of marketing data about their individual customers. I started looking at the potential to use that data for direct-marketing purposes. I had observed that a company such as Condé Nast in the United States, with a huge stable of magazines, was making $1.05 leveraging its customer data for every $1 that is made from advertising and sales of its magazines. It did this without selling any of its own data to other companies and so protected its brand and its relationship with its customers.

PBL had sixty-six magazines, Ticketek, Channel Nine, ninemsn and other web-based customers. Given my experience with targeted, permission-based marketing, I saw opportunities for PBL and many other companies, such as banks, insurance companies and large retailers, to be able to leverage their marketing data more effectively and appropriately, without compromising privacy considerations in any way.

I was unable to identify any Australian-based technology that was powerful enough to manage the huge number of databases that often existed within such large companies. I ended up in New York with an analyst from PBL, and we spent three weeks researching appropriate companies in the United States with US-based analysts. I ended up cold-calling the top three companies. Number two and three in Boston were not interested in an Australian presence, but with our visit to the biggest US company in this field, Acxiom, based in Little Rock, Arkansas, we struck gold.

The CEO and joint founder of this $2 billion a year revenue company was a larger-than-life character and entrepreneur, like the Packers. There were about 6000 people writing computer code— literally 5 acres of computer mainframes in climate-controlled facilities and a significant presence in Chicago and London—yet it was still not very hierarchical. The culture had considerable similarities to PBL.

I got on very well with the CEO, Charles Morgan, and I left there two days later with a handshake and a strong expression of interest in a joint venture. Within two months, we had a deal to form an Australian Acxiom company, a fifty-fifty joint venture between Acxiom and PBL.

Unexpectedly, I was asked to take on the CEO role for the set-up of this Australian arm of Acxiom. It was a totally consuming experience building a start-up company with national reach, getting to know the commercial landscape within the Australian direct-marketing industry, understanding the sophisticated technology that sat behind many of the solutions we were selling, gaining an effective knowledge of balance sheets and cash flow statements from a strictly commercial point of view, and working as part of a global company.

The 2 a.m. conference calls with colleagues in the United States and the frequent international travel played havoc with my body clock, combined with the pressure of building a business in an industry in which I hadn't had thirty years of commercial experience. Despite my nine years at the Liberal Party headquarters developing a 12 million–strong database, and commissioning the development of software to maintain, manage, enhance, analyse and share targeted groups with all of our campaign offices, this new pressure led to the morning depression hanging around longer on many days. Because I was running the company, I arranged not to have meetings before 9.30 a.m. unless I really had to. Nevertheless, I found the work enormously stimulating.

I turned fifty in 2001, and the election that year came and went. I realised that if I was going to try to win a parliamentary seat, it probably should have been that year, and not in another three years. Yet my Acxiom responsibilities meant I couldn't act on my ultimate ambitions, even if an opportunity had presented itself.

After the election, I shared my aspirations with the Packers. I had loved building up the business, but I couldn't get that excited about a long-term relationship with data. Also, Acxiom needed someone to run it who had strong industry and commercial experience and was going to make it their career. I stayed as chairman of the Australian arm of Acxiom and moved to an office with Australia's largest law firm, Minter Ellison, situated in the wonderful Renzo Piano–designed building in Phillip Street, Sydney.

It was Nick Greiner, the former New South Wales premier, who gave me the invaluable advice that led to me setting up in Minter Ellison. I am not a lawyer, and I explained I was looking for an office in a law firm with whom I could have a relationship but who would also let me run my own consultancy. He said such firms would not know in advance what work I might be able to do for them and so would be reluctant to put me on a retainer. He said, 'Just go and say to them you don't want a retainer; you want to be able to use an office, and maybe work for them as things occur'. It was a great strategy. An office is a marginal cost to a firm like Minter Ellison, with 1200 lawyers. My office was on the seventeenth floor, with extraordinary views down Sydney Harbour to the Heads.

The Managing Partner, Phil Clark, ensured my three years at Minter Ellison was a very valuable experience. I did little formal work with Minter Ellison but interacted extensively with their lawyers and participated in board lunches with the chairmen of their major client companies.

In my consulting practice, I sought to foster an advisory or facilitating role, rather than a lobbying role. I was selling my knowledge of politics, but because I had carried out such a large amount of strategic work, I ended up engaged in many projects that had no political component. When I first hung out my shingle, I had no idea of the extent of work that might come my way. Despite having two retainers from large companies I was still concerned about filling my diary. Those worries were soon erased.

On the second day, the phone rang at 11 a.m. and Tracey Winters, an executive working with Chevron in Western Australia, was enquiring about my availability and interest in being part of an investment team working on the huge Gorgon gas project off the state's north-west coast. Within a week I had spent two days in Perth being introduced to the project, and was then offered a twelve-month contract for two days a week.

In the end, twelve months turned into the full three years of my consulting practice. There were two investment teams working on the Gorgon project to determine the most profitable use of the gas. I was attached to the team that was investigating turning the gas into clean diesel—taking the gas back to CH4 and reconstituting the diesel molecule. This creates a product totally devoid of impurities, 40 per cent more fuel efficient than petrol, and ready to be distributed from the bowser system around Australia. It had the potential to supply close to 50 per cent of all of our transport fuel needs for more than a century. It was a truly exciting project. However, the LNG team ultimately won and I then moved to assist them, but clean diesel's day will come.

I had many other rewarding assignments, including working with Australia's thirty-nine vice chancellors for two years to help them deal with the big reforms that minister Brendan Nelson was making in higher education.

By the time I was consulting, Thaksin Shinawatra had succeeded in becoming Prime Minister of Thailand. I developed a range of Australian clients who were doing business in Thailand, including Pan Australia Resources, Oxiana, the Sydney Futures Exchange, and a couple of universities and entertainment groups. I spent up to a week a month in Bangkok for over two years. It was a valuable introduction to doing business in Asia.

Following a lot of political twists and turns in Thailand over recent years, Thaksin's sister, Yingluck Shinawatra, was elected in July 2011 as Thailand's first female Prime Minister, in a landslide victory.

I had projects with the big four accounting firms, a number of the law firms, PBL, Shell, Rio Tinto, BHP and other resource companies, large and small. During this period I was also a board member of Australia's largest consulting engineering company, Sinclair Knight Merz. I never ceased to be amazed by the world-leading innovation that the 6000 consulting engineers were driving.

My extracurricular activities involved being on the boards of the Menzies Research Centre, the Garvan Research Foundation, the

Big Brothers Big Sisters mentoring organisation, the Young Women's Christian Association (YWCA) business advisory panel, Chairman of the Australian Direct Marketing Association and a member of the Advisory Council, Strategic and Defence Studies Centre. While I was involved with a range of highly diverse and interesting projects, I still felt something was missing. I was giving advice, not calling the shots. I missed having responsibility, and the adrenaline and satisfaction that came with it. It was a privilege to work with the people and the companies, but those three years were a bit like a sabbatical in some respects, despite feeling that I was making a substantial contribution. I was itching to dedicate myself to the task of parliamentary life. That's when John Howard rang.

13

YES MINISTER

First John Howard rang. And then Peter Costello. It was 13 July 2004.

Dr David Kemp, a Cabinet minister and highly regarded member for the bayside seat of Goldstein in Melbourne, unexpectedly announced his intention to resign at the next election, due around October. He had held the seat since 1990.

In many ways I had almost moved on. I had been looking for a political opportunity since the previous 2001 election. We had been in Sydney for seven years, and given the nature of my work and travel, I had not been in a position to work up local party-member support in a particular seat. I was waiting for someone to retire; no-one did.

We were in the run up to the 2004 election, and I knew it was my last chance for a parliamentary opportunity. I was fifty-three and knew that, despite my experience, I would still need to serve my apprenticeship in parliament. It was my last chance. Faced with this seeming reality, I had started to negotiate a business commitment involving China, which would have locked me out of any opportunities beyond the 2004 election. But when John and

Peter asked if I was interested in standing for Goldstein, I said I would seriously think about it.

The year before, the Victorian Division had asked whether I was interested in considering the marginal seat of La Trobe in the Dandenongs. Maureen's sister lived near the bay in Melbourne, and her family was in country Victoria, so if we moved to Melbourne for a seat, I didn't think it was fair to live fifty minutes out of the city, where she knew no-one.

The Goldstein seat was a different proposition. Our boys Tom and Joe had finished school and were engaged in various work and study combinations. Our daughter Pip was finishing an interior design course. A move back to Melbourne was very inconvenient, but they were all in their twenties and reluctantly prepared to strike out on their own.

I had always been interested in a House of Representatives seat. People had occasionally sounded me out for a Senate seat, but I had always been more attracted to the chamber where government is formed. I wanted to try my hand at the senior jobs. I had worked with and observed senior Cabinet and Shadow Cabinet members, leaders, treasurers and the rest, and I felt I had the ability, experience and judgement to work well alongside them.

Halfway through my time as federal director, I had started to get a sense of what I could contribute in a parliamentary capacity on some of the big issues. By 2004, I had had significant exposure to indigenous communities, regional and rural Australia, the technical and tertiary sectors, small business, big business, the resources and energy sector, our ethnic communities, doing business in Asia, international trade negotiations, the media, the technology sector, mental health, programs directed at disadvantaged youth and more.

Originally I had associated politics with silver tongues, with the great stump orators. I am not blessed with such speaking skills, and

I thought they were a precondition for politics. But I discovered that, although I didn't have a flash style of communicating, I could get the message across, and people have suggested that I have a frank and thoughtful style. If I know my subject matter, I can convince people of my point of view.

I also knew I would like the electorate work. Constantly meeting people can be quite tiring, but I like that interaction. I am always fascinated by what motivates people and why they think what they think, and the best way to discover these things is to be in a social environment with them.

And I wanted the opportunity to influence policy decisions. I like decision-making; I like that responsibility and the excitement of challenges. Politics continues to offer lots of challenges on almost every issue. It is enormously satisfying to play a significant part in issues that affect millions of people.

I had three days to make a decision. In these situations, things move quickly. David announced his resignation on Tuesday, and I had until the Friday to decide in my own mind if I was serious about it. If I waited for another weekend, then a number of other candidates would be on the starting blocks.

I needed to meet all the key organisational people in the seat that weekend, when they were not at work. There are nearly 700 party members in Goldstein, and many have spent decades contributing their own time to running campaigns and supporting their local member—I needed to know that they were comfortable with me putting my hand up. I travelled to Melbourne and met forty people in two days.

It was important to convince them of my motivations and to assure them of my knowledge and empathy with Melbourne and Victoria, as I had never lived in that seat. Labor was already running the line, quite effectively, that the Liberals were looking to bring in a Sydneysider, that the Liberals were so bereft of talent that we had to import somebody.

There are still lots of people in the electorate who are surprised to learn that I was born in Melbourne, that it is where I spent the first twenty-eight years of my life, and that all my family are still in Victoria. The misconception that I come from Sydney is still hanging around seven years later, even among a few party supporters.

I had a good reception; people were fair and pleasant, and I enjoyed the conversations. On the plane trip back on the Sunday night, I thought if Maureen and the kids were happy with the change, I would commit. The seat of Goldstein is in a lovely part of Melbourne, not far from the CBD for meetings and not too far from the airport. Maureen was very supportive but not personally excited.

The first few months were difficult for all of us. I spent only two more nights at our home in Sydney. Maureen had to sell our Kirribilli house on her own and help the kids find alternative accommodation. As soon as I had made my decision, I could get away almost immediately, because of the way I had arranged my business affairs.

Within ten days, the other potential candidates had decided not to contest a preselection. This meant the party administration decided to bypass a preselection process and endorse me. Everyone had a sense the election was coming, so I started my local campaign immediately.

My job was to get myself established locally and make sure that there were no hiccups. Goldstein has always been held by the Liberal Party since Federation, usually with a margin of 7–8 per cent. As such there was an expectation that the Liberals would win, so there was a great interest in getting to know me.

I knew from experience that you might work as hard as you could for nine weeks meeting people and still only meet 5 per cent of the electorate, at best. This is where my direct-marketing experience came in.

I spent a considerable amount of time working out the best ways of communicating or introducing myself via direct marketing, and developing material that would be attractive to people. Much of it was non-political material about myself, informing them about my strengths and experience, and how I could effectively represent this local electorate.

I sought invitations through the local party members to a wide range of organisations. People were keen to hear my views. One day I was grilled by 130 members of the Independent Retirees for two and a half hours. I got around to every nursing home and bowling club I could. I visited schools, youth clubs, sailing clubs, football clubs and centres for the disabled. I went to many branch and community meetings, working hard to remember hundreds of names—not one of my strong points.

I rented an apartment just off Hampton Street in East Brighton and set up a campaign office just around the corner. My assistant, Margo Beales, had been with me a long time, and as I was still winding up my business interests, she kindly came and assisted with these commitments and the campaign. She was invaluable.

I can't stand living by myself. I've been in hotel rooms all my life, and I still can't sit in them, even if I have got a good book to read. I'm either sleeping, working or down at the bar having a drink, reading my book or speaking to other hotel guests. I need people around me. Everyone was very good to me, but I didn't have any friends around. Then a great university friend of mine, Chris Grieve, came to Melbourne from his property near Wangaratta to support me for the last five weeks of the campaign. Chris stayed with his mother and helped with much of the correspondence and queries from the public at our campaign office. And just as important, he kept me laughing for the five weeks with his wicked sense of humour. It made a big difference to my frame of mind because I was anxious about whether I had done the right thing by Maureen and the kids.

We had teams of people out letterboxing. We targeted family areas and produced a brochure on the Greens. There was a fear the Liberal voters would drift to the Greens because there were seventeen environmental groups in my electorate. It is such a beautiful part of Melbourne, with the bay and the parks, and many people who live in Goldstein have strong environmental interests. I produced pamphlets that exposed a lot of the other policies that the Greens had on drugs and injecting rooms, policies that most Liberals would find abhorrent and reject. So we put those pamphlets around in the last week in strong Liberal areas.

I felt particularly despondent in the mornings during that period. I think it was a combination of my usual condition, being on my own and trying to think through the consequences for my family. I found the King Club pool in Sandringham, where Michael Klim is involved, and went there each morning at 6 a.m. to swim. The noise and atmosphere were good for me. After a shower, I would head to a local coffee shop where I had got to know the owners. I'd buy the papers; I'd be saying 'Hello' to all and sundry, and by the time I got to the office, it would be 8.30 a.m. and my confidence would be starting to return.

I personally raised $70 000 for the campaign, and the party had already collected quite a bit of money. In a marginal seat, more than $400 000 can be spent, while in safer, established seats, as little as $70 000 could be needed if someone is really well known. I needed to spend more than the usual amount for safe seats to compensate for not having lived in the area.

Mark Latham was leader of the ALP, and by the time the campaign had begun, John Howard had started to get his measure. I had felt confident for three or four months that Latham was beatable, and that conviction only increased as the election campaign rolled on; his performance deteriorated by the day.

On polling night we felt pretty confident from as early as 7 p.m. Maureen and the kids came down, and we were in a function room at Milanos in Brighton. A few hundred party members were there. You couldn't really hear the commentary on the various flat-screen TVs around the room because of the conversations and excitement. I gave up trying to assess things; in any event, it was clear that I had won. As it turned out, it was by the second-largest margin ever in the history of the seat. The party was also heading for a big win, almost back to the 1996 record level. It was hugely satisfying, but it took me twelve months not to feel like an interloper in Goldstein.

Once I was elected and Canberra sittings had begun, Peter Costello warned me, 'You've got no appreciation of what it's like when you're in full throttle at the dispatch box at Question Time and you can't hear a word that you're saying because of the noise coming at you from the other side'. He said it's a special art to put nuance in your voice when you can't hear it.

The first time I understood what Peter had been talking about was just before 2 p.m. (when Question Time starts) some eight or nine months later. People were pouring into the chamber, and I had about four minutes of speaking time left on an industrial relations Bill relating to WorkChoices, an issue of obsession for Labor. As all the MPs entered, I started going for it in front of the full 150 members, decrying what a miserable mob they were on the other side of the Chamber and why no-one should have anything to do with them. They were all screaming at me, full throttle. Peter was right.

I spent a lot of time working on my maiden speech. I wanted to use the opportunity to sum up my philosophy, and to discuss why I wanted to be in parliament and my expectations of the job. It was a defining moment. Maiden speeches are always referred to. I had to convey my priorities and the values that were important to me, and I also wanted to use the speech as a reference point in the future, so I would be able to see whether my views had changed or if I had drifted from what I initially believed. I put a lot of time into preparing it.

A constituent and public-presentation expert, Tina Owens, contacted me and offered 'help at any stage'. I didn't know Tina, but I gave her a copy of the draft of my maiden speech. A few days later, it came back with a letter tearing it to shreds; mainly, it was boring. After feeling offended for twenty-four hours, I read Tina's suggestions for significant structural change and started to see her point. I did some major reworking.

There was a focus on comparing the maiden speeches that year— Malcolm Turnbull, Peter Garrett and myself included. The gallery in the House of Representatives was full of Malcolm's supporters who had come down from his electorate in the eastern suburbs of Sydney to hear his speech. Coincidentally, Mark Latham was speaking about another Bill before Malcolm and I got to our feet.

I felt that I had done the best job I could. Then Malcolm gave his address, which was an excellent, well-crafted speech of almost poetic observations of his seat and Bondi. The next day, the *Financial Review* ran a piece by journalist Laura Tingle headed, 'Malcolm Grins, Robb Wins'. It pays to take advice. Tina has continued to help me, as well as giving encouragement. She has analysed my strengths—honesty, frankness, calmness—and reminded me that people only want to see what you are. That is the most effective way to communicate.

It helped greatly, as I was trying to manage my still unconfronted morning problem, which was starting to sap my self-belief. The mornings were becoming more inconvenient once I turned fifty.

It took longer each day before I popped out of that state of indecision: 9 a.m., 9.30 a.m., some days 10.30 a.m., and even into the afternoon.

I started my parliamentary career on the backbench focusing on economics. After eight months I was made chairman of a taskforce promoting WorkChoices. In year two I was appointed Parliamentary Secretary to the Minister for Immigration and Multicultural Affairs. I was promoted to the ministry in my third year, as Minister for Vocational Education.

Despite these excellent opportunities I was, as always, impatient. I think, in hindsight, that if I had been elevated too quickly, then some of my problems with depression would have materialised sooner, perhaps in a damaging way, and it might have been much more difficult to come back to public life.

14

HOWARD'S END

I can claim to never having been bored in my seven years of parliamentary life. During the first six years (or two terms), I had five different portfolio responsibilities. I was paddling hard.

Early in my first year, I became chairman of a newly formed Coalition taskforce to explain and promote WorkChoices, our new industrial relations policy. After one month, it was already attracting a storm of Labor and union protest. I travelled across Australia addressing many organisations, and talking to local media. The policy had taken everyone by surprise: the party room and the electorate. The first hurdle faced was that very few people had a sense of what the existing industrial relations problems were that WorkChoices sought to address. To successfully introduce major changes, first you have to show people that there is a problem that needs to be solved. This hadn't been done. With the strong economy and low unemployment, people were confused about the reason for the changes. They were therefore vulnerable to a union–Labor campaign suggesting sinister motives.

HOWARD'S END

The policy package had two major weaknesses: the removal of the no-disadvantage test, which made it difficult to answer the question, 'Can you guarantee that no-one will be worse off?', and the exemption from unfair dismissal laws for businesses up to 100 employees instead of the previous 20-employee limit.

Ironically, Labor retained many elements of the WorkChoices legislation, despite restoring unprecedented power to the unions. They have turned WorkChoices into UnionChoices.

Of equal interest is that WorkChoices was still effectively operating through the GFC before Labor's changes came into effect, and provided the flexibility for employers who were hard hit to reduce working hours rather than having to put people off. This has never been possible in previous recessions, such as that of 1990–91, when hundreds of thousands of people were laid off, and the number of unemployed reached one million. As such, the impact of the GFC on working families was much less than it might have been, and once the worst was over, the hours worked per week jumped back to pre-GFC levels quite quickly.

As Parliamentary Secretary, I was responsible for multicultural affairs, the settlement of refugees, asylum-seeker detention centres, family-reunion visas and citizenship. I arrived in the job at the time of the Cronulla riots and the subsequent focus on Muslim issues, and later the Lebanese–Israeli war.

My many meetings with imams and other Muslim leaders around Australia, and my introduction to many Australian Muslim communities, only hardened my view of the fundamental need to focus on getting new arrivals to Australia into work if they are to integrate quickly and effectively.

The Australian Turkish community, for example, has long been successfully integrated into the broader Australian community, and they are not identified by their religion, and yet they are the biggest Muslim community in Australia. On arrival they moved quickly into the workforce, and everything else fell into place.

By contrast, the Lakemba Lebanese Muslim community, led by the controversial Sheikh Hilali, arrived during the 1970s Lebanese war, expecting to return home after the war ended. It never happened. Most failed to get employment, and now, more than thirty years later, they remain isolated—almost an island within Sydney's west—with very high unemployment among the first and second generation.

I took responsibility for the dismantling of the Muslim Community Reference Group because I saw it as both unrepresentative and a vehicle for further alienating the broader Australian community, to everyone's disadvantage. I convened a meeting of Australia's 100 imams and stated as bluntly as I could that the controversy and the concern about radicalism was 'your problem, not the problem of the broader Australian community', and that they had to accept prime responsibility for fixing it. We could help, but they had to lead. I came to strongly respect many of the Muslim community leaders, such as Sheikh Fehmi, who took over from Sheikh Hilali as the mufti of Australia.

I place much of the blame for the absence of any direction in the Lakemba community at Hilali's feet, with his constant refrain over the years that his Lakemba flock were morally superior to the millions of non-Muslims around them. It served to justify their excessive dependence on welfare, which worked against their integration into the Australian community.

I was responsible for initially advocating, and ultimately getting through Cabinet, the need for the citizenship test. I was sorry not to remain working on it through to its ultimate design. I was motivated to introduce such a test after seeing so many refugee women who couldn't speak English.

It was a flashback to my teenage years in Reservoir, where there was a large Italian population who had migrated after World War II. Their lives were all about providing an education for their kids, many of whom were my schoolfriends. A lot of their mothers couldn't speak English, even though they might have been here for fifteen years or more. Their husbands were in the workforce and soon learnt English. The kids had to interpret for their mothers. In some cases, their mothers still can't speak English, and now the tragedy is that they can't speak to their grandchildren, or great-grandchildren, because the children can't speak Italian. It is very sad.

At the time I was parliamentary secretary, Maureen was doing volunteer work at the Monash Medical Centre with expectant mothers who were newly arrived refugees from Africa, Afghanistan and other countries. She remarked that most of these women couldn't speak English. They were striking women with a lot going for them, but because of their lack of English, many were timid and apprehensive. Most of their husbands could speak English because they were working. It was history repeating itself. I strongly believed that these women, and thousands like them, could get much more out of life in Australia if they could speak English. There were free English-language classes all over the country.

I decided that requiring a basic level of English competence to get citizenship would provide an enormous incentive to learn English. I floated the idea in a speech at the Sydney Institute, and within weeks there was a massive increase in the number of immigrant and refugee women enrolling in English-language classes. The proposal got a lot of coverage in the media, and then false rumours started that even new citizens might have their passports taken away from them if they didn't speak English. So even people with citizenship started going to English-language classes. I was delighted.

At the start of my third year, the election year, I was appointed Minister for Vocational Education. With skill shortages emerging as the mining boom gathered pace, we were moving quickly on many fronts to dramatically increase the number of people who were completing technical training. One very exciting and effective initiative was John Howard's decision to reinstate stand-alone technical colleges for years 11 and 12, with a curriculum that ensured graduates not only achieved a Year 12 certificate, but would also be well into their apprenticeship for their chosen trade. Twenty-one of these colleges were complete, and six were well on the way, by the time of the election.

The colleges were an outstanding success. For the first time in their lives, many of the students felt that their particular talents were being recognised and fostered. Their confidence, self-esteem and enthusiasm rose accordingly.

Despite the extraordinary success, Labor vowed to stop this program because of a deal they did with the education unions, who feared losing control of secondary education. Subsequently, Labor has either placed the schools within the Catholic or independent schools system, or starved others of any growth potential.

The year also taught me another lesson in the failings of a highly centralised management system in education. Australia's TAFE colleges represent 76 per cent of the infrastructure involved in technical education. Yet great disparities in the effectiveness of these organisations exist around Australia. In the 1990s, Jeff Kennett, as Premier of Victoria, gave a large measure of autonomy to those running the Victorian TAFE colleges, including allowing them to reinvest any of the profits they made. By 2007, the differences between Victorian TAFE colleges and most others around Australia, especially in New South Wales, were profound. A range of business and educational partnerships, both here and overseas, along with the flexible delivery of training packages for business (either on campuses or at the business enterprise), pathways to degrees and much more have led to the provision of world-class technical education at colleges like the Holmesglen and Box Hill TAFEs. While some states are now making tentative moves in that direction, New South Wales still requires ministerial approval for the CEO of any TAFE to buy an air ticket to fly outside Australia on business. Some of these TAFEs are businesses turning over more than $100 million. It beggars belief.

So I had plenty to engage me, and I learnt a great deal being part of John Howard's team. One of John's great strengths is his ability to speak off the cuff, aided by an extraordinary memory. Often before he had to speak, he would discuss the potential structure of the speech and the key issues to be covered. He would write down several dot points on a piece of paper. He would ask who in the audience needed to be acknowledged, and their title or claim to fame. He'd commit possibly six or eight names, and titles, to memory. Then he would rise to speak, invariably without missing a beat. Often he would not need to pull out his dot points. Presumably, he could see them in his mind's eye, along with the substance of the issues that sat behind each dot point. It was a wonderful gift, and John made the most of it. But his greatest skill was to distil the core of a problem or opportunity into language that people could understand, and then stay with that message consistently, in words accessible to everybody, until the issue had been won or lost.

Despite such skills, experience and outstanding achievements, however, there always comes a time when some new blood at the top is desirable. It seems that many leaders eventually feel so in control of the job that they don't need to listen anymore. With John, that became more and more evident as his fourth term progressed.

No doubt John thought he could win. He had a huge victory against Latham in 2004; it was the fourth election he had fought in a row, and he nearly took the Coalition back to the dizzy heights of 1996, in terms of seats won. It was a phenomenal effort, but the result created a sense in the party room that no-one had the right to question his political judgement. Many, including myself, were thinking, I consider myself experienced, but who am I? Here is a guy who's won four elections, and not only that but he buried his opponent in the last one.

I suspect we were somewhat blinded by the extent of his success in that 2004 election for a while. Possibly many of us stopped giving our political views as forthrightly as we might have given them previously, and perhaps John himself was overly influenced by his own success. Whatever the reason, many colleagues, especially the class of '96, assumed he would get us back on top. Most of us thought that John had a cunning plan in there somewhere, and it would emerge. We were wrong.

In terms of preferred prime minister, John was still in a reasonable position fifteen months out from the election. Then the letter Ian McLachlan had carried around in his wallet for all those years, supposedly recording an agreement for John Howard to hand over to Peter Costello, was leaked. Experienced journalist Glenn Milne splashed it all over the front pages of the Sunday papers.

John denied the agreement. Peter effectively called him a liar. Both men, and their supporters, were forced back into their corners, snarling. John said he was staying. Peter was a long way from having the numbers to successfully challenge him. It wasn't our greatest week for unity.

It was something of a tipping point. Our fortunes in the polls, slowly but surely, deteriorated. By early December, we were 10 points behind. As such, Kim Beazley must have felt badly jilted to then face a challenge, and ousting, by Kevin Rudd.

In politics the change of leadership comes, more often than not, with blood on the floor. In a way, it's almost necessary, because the only way people can really judge if a person is strong enough to be leader is to see whether that person can stare down an incumbent, and whether he or she is tough enough to go through that exercise.

John Howard's great strength is his determination. But just as I learnt with Paul Keating, strengths can also be weaknesses—two sides of the same coin. John's resolve, determination, persistence and strength of character under pressure also turned out to be weaknesses, because all of those qualities meant it would be very hard for him to give up anything. Someone was always going to have to take the leadership away from him, and when Peter Costello wouldn't, no-one else was positioned to.

Who knows what would have happened if we had moved to Peter? We would have given the electorate a choice, and Peter is a very formidable politician. At the very least, we would have won a lot more seats and put Kevin Rudd under pressure. He didn't face any pressure for three years until Tony Abbott came along.

Peter had positioned himself on all those symbolic issues—'Sorry' and Kyoto—and he was a new generation but with tremendous experience. He offered a whole lot of 'new' with a whole lot of 'old'. It would have highlighted Kevin's inexperience. But I think this was realised too late. We were in freefall, and we hadn't gained any traction against Kevin through the first half of 2007.

Everyone is always inclined to think that the current campaign will play out like the previous campaign. Labor feared John had something up his sleeve, and there was complacency on our side that he did, but by July it was clear there was no rabbit; the hat was empty.

The polling in late August and early September 2007, some two to three months before the expected election, convinced everyone we were heading for a calamity in terms of potential seat losses. In fact, the 4 September Newspoll, four days before John was to host world leaders at the Sydney APEC meeting, saw Labor jump to a

59–41 lead. It was clear we were going to lose. My focus turned to protecting as much as we could, so at least we would be in a better position the next time round.

Alexander Downer met with colleagues secretly on the Thursday night after John initiated some sort of review of his position by the Cabinet. On the Friday, Alexander was to report back to John and Janette Howard what their colleagues had concluded.

Being in the outer ministry I was unaware of any of this. I rang Alexander that Friday morning thinking he was the best-placed person to give me advice about John's frame of mind. I wasn't in Cabinet, but I'd been campaign director in the 1990s. It gave me some authority, and it wasn't improper or impertinent for me to get involved. Alexander briefed me on what had transpired over the previous three or four days. He said the sense was that John should go, but it was John's decision; the Cabinet wouldn't insist that he go. That seemed weak to me, but there was a rationale behind it—the Cabinet thought that the party organisation would go into meltdown if the Cabinet moved against John. I gave Alexander my view that John had a responsibility to either limit the damage or give us a chance by standing aside. I felt that it would be best if Cabinet requested it, otherwise it would look like John was running away. Alexander asked if he could pass my thoughts onto John, which I presume he did.

There were still a lot of discussions going on over the weekend and even on the Sunday night. I thought there was a prospect that, on the Monday, John would pull up stumps. The issue had leaked to the papers, and over that weekend quite a few of my own electorate members rang expressing their outrage that John could be dumped by his Cabinet. For historical reasons my electorate was quite pro-Howard. I could see where the Cabinet was coming from: there would have been meltdown.

On the Monday morning we were back in parliament; John didn't resign, and there was heated debate for a couple of days. He was saying how determined he was, and that he would fight any challenge, and Peter Costello went back into his burrow.

However, on the Wednesday night, John was interviewed on *The 7:30 Report* by Kerry O'Brien and, in the middle of it, announced that he wouldn't see the next term out, that he would retire during the next term. It was a bizarre announcement, and I felt it severely damaged us because he had effectively labelled himself as a lame duck prime minister even before the election was held.

I was back in my electorate on the Thursday night, when I coincidentally had two electorate functions where I caught up with 140 of my members, and certainly the most active ones. Many of those who had rung me the weekend before, to tell me how outraged they were by the rumours about Cabinet moving against John, were now saying, 'You know, I think Costello would do quite well against Rudd in the debates'. They had moved on.

Once John had said he was going to leave, people instantly moved to the next person. The king is dead, long live the king. They weren't angry; they were thinking, He's moved on in his mind. If he's saying he's going to retire at some time in the next three years, it will be sooner rather than later, and that's where his head's at. Good on him—he's done a great job—so time for Costello.

It couldn't get any more definitive. It was the worst of all worlds. After talking to a few colleagues, I felt I had to do something, that it still wasn't too late. There was another week in parliament. I decided I had to speak to John directly. I rang Tony Nutt, who was John's Chief of Staff, and asked to see John the next night in Canberra. A couple of hours later, he asked if I could be at the Lodge at 8 p.m. on the Sunday night.

When I got there, John said, 'There's no staff around tonight; would you like a cup of tea?' So we sat in the front sitting room sipping our tea. John makes a lovely cup of tea.

As had always been the way between us, it was a non-acrimonious discussion; it was all very professional. I spent half an hour passing on what had happened in the last two weeks from my perspective, and my conclusions. I said that I thought things had demonstrably changed again on the Wednesday night, and that party members would no longer go into meltdown if Cabinet requested him to resign. John then spent half an hour telling me why Peter Costello wouldn't do as well as he would. I listened intently, but I found none of it convincing. Everything he said had been aired over the previous weeks, and I didn't agree.

John said, 'Are you asking me to resign?' I saw it as no different from a company where the chairman has to respect the wishes of his or her board. I responded, 'No, I'm not asking you to resign. I think that would then be presented as you running away from a perceived loss, and that's not fair to you, given what you've done for the country and for the party, and you couldn't be expected to do that'. I said, 'You need to have your Cabinet ask you to resign. It's not a reflection on your contribution; it's just life'.

I told John that I thought there was still time to make the change, and that I was going to see his Cabinet ministers the next day and would seek to convince them to reconvene, given that circumstances had changed. John's announcement of his intended mid-term retirement increased the likelihood that Cabinet would move against him. He simply said, 'OK'. I think he was also thinking, Good luck. You'll need it.

I hadn't told anybody I was going to see John. I went back to my apartment and made appointments with all my Cabinet colleagues. I had had ministerial responsibility for two years, one as a parliamentary secretary and one as a minister, and almost all of the Cabinet members had been through the 1996 campaign when I was Federal Director and Campaign Director. They saw me as an equal, certainly on political matters, and I got a good hearing.

I got to almost all of them. I didn't see Tony Abbott because I thought he was committed to John, even though he had been a bit ambivalent the week before. I saw Alexander Downer; he thought John should go. I only missed one or two people, and I thought there was a real prospect that I had laid the groundwork for change.

There was another poll the next day; it was a fortnight after the poll that had resulted in 59–41, Labor leading. If it had stayed at 59–41, or even been 58–42, I think there was a real chance that Cabinet would have been spurred into action, without the fear of a party meltdown. As it turned out, the poll returned to 55–45 and many said the recovery was on! Yet it only got worse for us until well into the election; it got a little bit closer towards the end.

I saw several of John Howard's colleagues, and they didn't have the stomach for dealing with the issue, because it looked like the polls were moving. There was a mood change to, 'Ah, that was an aberration, and now he still will pull a rabbit out of the hat'. After that, there was a sense of resignation that that's the way it was going to be. So that was it. I was in a hurry to be part of some big decisions for our country. The prospect of being thrown into Opposition after just three years was soul destroying.

John and I never talked about that conversation, and he has never shown any animosity towards me because of it. It was politics, and we had a very mature conversation. I assumed he had a sense of the respect I had for what he'd achieved for Australia.

15

A NEW ERA

I did take a chance coming in to a government that, at the time, had been in power for seven years. And the disrupted lead-up to the campaign meant we were forever on the back foot. We never gained momentum, and morale was flat.

As always, by election night I had the flu. I was in Canberra appearing on the Channel 7 panel at the national tally room with Labor's Mark Arbib, former Queensland premier Peter Beattie, the National Party's Barnaby Joyce and Jeff Kennett. Barnaby was in pretty good form, as was Jeff, but it felt to me like a total waste of time. I wasn't well, and all I wanted to do was to be with my family and electorate supporters, having a quiet drink before an early night. The result was obvious so early on that it felt like we were just filling in three hours.

I caught a plane back to Melbourne the next morning, arriving home at noon. I was really tired and fluey; I lay down on the couch looking forward to a snooze for a couple of hours. I assumed Peter Costello would take over, and that I would worry about what was ahead of us over the next week or two.

About an hour later, the phone rang and the party's Federal Director, Brian Loughnane, said, 'I think you should turn on the TV and watch Sky in about ten minutes', without telling me what was happening. Peter Costello came on, with his wife Tanya, and said that he was going to leave politics.

The last thing I felt like was getting immediately back into the fray. I had been based at campaign headquarters for the thirty-three days of the campaign as the campaign spokesperson. Given my morning ailment, it had been a tough five weeks, as I had been campaigning at night and weekends in my own electorate. Nevertheless, I thought it would be on for young and old, and I wanted to at least position myself and show my intentions. Malcolm Turnbull had already declared that he was running for leader.

I rang a couple of guys and told them I was interested in running for deputy. By 2.15 p. m., with their encouragement, I was already on the phone making calls and putting forward my pitch. Brendan Nelson also declared that he was running for leader, but Julie Bishop didn't declare until the next day. That was the smarter move, because the vote wasn't until Tuesday, two days away.

For the next couple of days I was on the phone nonstop, working very hard on the calls because there is no point being half-hearted if you have put your hand up.

The major focus was on the two prospective leaders. The Right came to see me and said that they were going to support Brendan Nelson, and if he got up, they would support Julie Bishop, because they thought she would project an important image for us, as Julia Gillard was Deputy Prime Minister. But they told me that if Malcolm got up, they would shift their vote to me, guaranteeing about nine votes. They did not trust Malcolm and wanted me by his side if he won.

Brendan won, and with the Right's support Julie easily won the deputy job. Brendan offered me Finance, which I should have taken, but I thought there would be less chance to engage with the public in that portfolio. In the end I got Foreign Affairs, which I found very stimulating.

Foreign Affairs probably delayed me from confronting the morning issue because it didn't demand a lot of media work. I had always taken a keen interest in the subject, so I took to it quickly and really engaged with the issues. I tried to just focus on one or two issues, because Kevin Rudd was seen to be such an expert in foreign affairs, even though he started off by offending the Japanese by sending a frigate to follow Japan's whaling activities, and then didn't visit Japan—our largest trading partner—for nearly five months after winning the prime ministership.

Brendan's twelve months as leader were really tough. Kevin and Labor were riding high, and Brendan faced endless destabilisation from Malcolm and his supporters. It was unrelenting. I greatly admired his fortitude and decency. Unfortunately he wasn't gaining popularity in the electorate.

Malcolm has one of the biggest brain boxes I've come across. I suspect Kevin's is not far off it either. Their intelligence means they see every side of every issue, so much so that it can interfere with their judgement. It is highly entertaining to spend time with Malcolm, and in the main, he doesn't take himself too seriously. Many people would find that an odd thing to say, but there are two Malcolms in a way: the one that's easygoing, inquisitive, concerned, interesting, interested and entertaining; and then there's the ambitious Malcolm, who wants to get somewhere, either with a deal or in politics, and can be totally ruthless, intransigent, bullying, unpleasant and with a measure of self-belief that I've never observed in anybody else.

I remember going into Malcolm's office at PBL on a number of occasions during 1985 and you couldn't see the floor for scrunched-up bits of paper. Malcolm was sitting there in the middle of it, like a man floating on an ocean of crumpled paper. He was oblivious to it, and I made some comment about the fact that I couldn't see the floor. Malcolm replied, 'There are too many secrets in here to leave the door unlocked for the cleaner'.

When Malcolm took over, I wanted to get back into the economic area because I thought that would be the ground on which the election would be fought. Joe Hockey was ultimately appointed Shadow Treasurer by Malcolm after Julie Bishop stumbled, and I had to settle for a new portfolio—Climate Change, Infrastructure and Council of Australian Governments (COAG).

While I had my sights on other portfolios, this portfolio certainly brought me back into the thick of things, especially with climate change. I had done a couple of years of strategic work on climate change when I was consulting, and was familiar with the scientific debate and some of the arguments around the supposed solutions.

Early in my career as an economist, I teamed up with two scientists off and on over a period of eighteen months to two years, evaluating the scientific techniques and relevance of the research being carried out at various agricultural research stations. My background in agricultural science, economics and statistical technique gave me a good grounding. I had also written computer models for commercial purposes over a two-year period, and commissioned a wide range of modelling work over eight years at the NFF and nine years at the federal secretariat.

In our investigations of agricultural research, I came across a lot of good science associated with very poor statistical technique, and I saw some scientists whose projects were dictated more by what could keep them near their 400- or 500-acre properties, which were fifteen to twenty minutes from the research station.

With climate change, I observed similar trends, and I had formed the view that there should be no alarmists and no deniers—that everyone should be a sceptic somewhere along the continuum between both extremes. I still hold that view.

The potential for error remains enormous, and the climate change modelling contains many heroic assumptions, given the huge range of variables involved. And the religious and moral overtones are an insult and are highly counterproductive.

I had half an hour with Hewlett Packard's former CEO Mark Hurd two years ago and asked him what his company was doing about carbon dioxide emissions. Hewlett Packard, a $75 billion business, is a huge power user with massive data centres around the world. Mark said, 'We don't talk much about CO2. However, six years ago we took a board decision to reduce our usage of power. By a thousand different ways we have halved our power usage'. And he said, 'By the way, in the process, we have halved the CO2 emissions we are responsible for'. This is a 'no regrets', direct-action approach.

Any policy pursued in the short to medium term should be a 'no regrets', direct-action policy, which achieves outcomes that are worthwhile irrespective of the scientific outcome, such as Hewlett Packard's improved energy efficiency. Such approaches don't lock Australia into policies that create huge future property rights issues and competitive disadvantages if the rest of the world, especially our major competitors, don't follow our lead with an emissions trading scheme.

China is following a 'no regrets', direct-action policy as they clean up much of the environmental degradation caused over generations, and as they improve the efficiency of so many of their manufacturing practices.

That is why, in the end, I so strongly opposed Labor's emissions trading scheme (ETS) policy. It is very bad policy, and it is being pursued again for largely political reasons. If you set out to design the most bureaucratic, high-taxing, interventionist, government-directed, socialistic policy, Labor's ETS would fit the bill. To suggest it is a pure market system is a joke. The potential for scamming is enormous.

There are even other ways of constructing an emissions trading scheme that are far less taxing and interventionist, where large carbon dioxide emitters still face the same carbon price, which the government has refused point blank to debate and consider. The community can smell the manipulation and self-interest, and is responding accordingly.

Climate change policy is a huge issue, demanding a significant amount of work to understand the complexities and to discover if there are alternative schemes. That meant constant meetings, lots of speeches and lots of press conferences. I had about eighty-five companies or organisations that I was dealing with, and I met with many of them regularly. Some days I would have seven meetings with CEOs, and four of them might be before midday. My morning malaise was lasting later into the day, and often I did not feel confident until eleven or twelve o'clock, which was so tedious. I'd really be working hard to engage properly and it was increasingly frustrating and difficult, and I was concerned about the impact on my effectiveness.

In these meetings I would be talking to myself saying, 'Pull yourself together, just concentrate'. I just needed the adrenaline to kick in, but those meetings were not confrontational. I was very practised in those situations, so I could still carry the meeting off, but I was acting and not feeling self-assured.

When I entered parliamentary life in 2004, people would ask, 'Are you enjoying politics again?' and 'Are you enjoying being a Member of Parliament?' I would always say, 'I find it enormously satisfying'. I would consciously avoid saying, 'I am enjoying it', because I wasn't. I was getting satisfaction because I was achieving things, but I was seldom enjoying myself. All that has now changed.

The anxiety was drifting into the afternoons, especially with media performances, but I still wouldn't admit to myself that I had depression. Since my mid-thirties, I had often bought books on how to think positively. I would never pick up a book on depression, because that was tantamount to admitting I had that affliction. Ironically, when I finally confronted my depression and then looked at some books on depression, many of the techniques being suggested were not dissimilar to the suggestions in the 'positive thinking' books.

I could always sleep, through all the years of campaigning and all the crises in politics. That's what probably got me through as I got older and had more responsibility, and as the morning problem was becoming increasingly evident. I could always say to myself, Well you just had six hours of solid sleep; it's going to be fine.

I deeply wish I had confronted my depression earlier. I can't help but think how much more effective I might have been, but better late than never.

16

AN ACT OF TREACHERY

I had gone public and stepped down from Shadow Cabinet, but I was trying to assist Malcolm Turnbull and Ian Macfarlane with climate change matters ahead of the negotiations with the government. Kevin Rudd had gone to the election saying they would introduce an emissions trading scheme, and Malcolm was saying at every opportunity that we had to support a version of it or else the government would call a double dissolution. We never discussed the science, and I was increasingly of the view that the ETS was deeply flawed and very bad policy.

My trip to Washington and Beijing in July 2009 had convinced me that neither the United States nor China would embrace an ETS for a decade or more, if ever. Going it alone seemed madness, involving a tax on our great strength, energy and resources.

At this time I was suffering from depression 24/7 as a side effect of the drug Lexapro. It was soon after that I switched to the drug I am still on today, Pristiq. I didn't feel constant depression as a side effect, but I felt very dopey. I would want to sleep a lot of the time.

I would find myself nodding off, and yet, irritatingly, I couldn't sleep at night for the first time in my life.

Often I wasn't getting to sleep until 5.30 a.m., only to wake up again at 6.30 a.m. and head off to help Malcolm and Ian. However, I increasingly realised I was just being humoured; they weren't really interested in the range of concerns and other options I presented. I would arrange briefings for them by experts, and there would be surreptitious smirks of dismissal between Malcolm and his senior staff. I was feeling really bad on the new drug and decided to go back to my electorate, leaving them to it.

My staff were still helping them though, which is how I discovered that in the first round of negotiations over the changes that should be made to the government's ETS, about three of the issues I considered fundamental to the Coalition's position were jettisoned. The Minister for Climate Change and Water, Penny Wong, said, 'Under no circumstance will I take those things to Cabinet'. Malcolm just said, 'OK, next', and they moved on.

I didn't see a lot of Malcolm because parliament wasn't sitting and I was dealing with the new drug, but whenever I did, he would say, 'We are still fighting'. When I would query him about particulars, knowing full well that he had already caved in, he would reply, 'Oh no, we are really hanging in for that still'. Malcolm and Ian kept saying that no final decisions would be made until the last few days, and claimed they were still defending all our positions.

We had commissioned further independent modelling research, which, if made public during the negotiations, would have strengthened our hand considerably. The results were kept from my colleagues and the media and given to Penny Wong. I was dumbstruck. It was not a negotiation. I suspect it was a series of discussions as to how to make it look as though the Coalition had had a big win and the government had got an ETS.

At 4 p.m. the day before the Shadow Cabinet and partyroom meetings, unbeknown to Malcolm and Ian, I saw a confidential copy of what was going to be presented at the meetings for an ultimate decision. It was a total sell-out, but it was so cleverly crafted that it would look, to the less informed, like we'd won the lottery in the negotiations.

I was furious. I got all of my speeches and all the speeches that Malcolm had given through the year on the issues of an ETS. I worked in my apartment until 11 p.m., researching, calling people for details, and prepared an explanation of the huge holes in the Coalition's proposition in a way that I thought my colleagues would understand.

It is an enormously complicated scheme and is hard to comprehend. Very few people do. There is also much language designed to confuse people. 'Price on carbon', for example, is not on carbon at all; it's on carbon dioxide. Nor is it a price; it's a tax—for some people it is a subsidy, and to everyone else it's a tax. This issue is full of these euphemisms to mislead people.

Some people tried to get me to go to Shadow Cabinet to help them decipher it, people such as Nick Minchin, Tony Abbott, Eric Abetz and some of the Nationals. I declined and said I was not a member of Shadow Cabinet. I was on leave from it. I didn't want to show my hand. I knew that if Malcolm had any forewarning before the partyroom meeting, I would have found myself speaking last. I had been trying to get the Coalition to hold off making a deal until we saw what happened at Copenhagen, and to see what the United States was going to do.

Malcolm dismissed all this and insisted the government's Bill be passed before the summer recess. I decided I was battling a clever and well-orchestrated campaign. It was the biggest structural adjustment these politicians would ever face in terms of its impact on our economy, and the people making the decision on our side of politics were going to hear the results of the negotiations, have a 45-minute explanation, then a debate and then vote on it. It was cunning, and irresponsible in the extreme. I knew that if I didn't say anything, there was no-one else equipped to challenge the proposal, and I had just spent a year of my life getting on top of the subject.

The presentation to Shadow Cabinet early on Tuesday went for fifty minutes, with ten minutes of questions. Given the 'Pollyanna' view presented, the members of Shadow Cabinet felt they were left with no new arguments to oppose it.

I don't know whether I was expected at the partyroom meeting, and even though I turned up, people didn't necessarily think that I would speak, because they didn't know whether I was well enough. When the debate started, it was clear that most people were going to speak. I put up my hand early to get on the list of speakers, but clearly there was a predetermined speaking order. I don't know where Malcolm put me on the list, but it was running one for, one against. It was the few enthusiastic ones to start with and then it was one each way. The psychology had been thought through, but it was clear that it was going to go on for many hours.

For the first half-hour after the presentation, everyone was standing up and really saying what they had said all year. It was as if the morning presentation or the whole negotiation had not happened, because no-one understood enough; they just gave their longstanding positions. It was a hollow debate, and you could see people just going through the motions because they couldn't assess the result of the negotiations; it looked like it was preordained and the deal was going to get up.

After about half an hour, Michael Ronaldson, a friend and colleague from Victoria and one of Malcolm's lieutenants, came from the back of the room. I was in a row near the front. He lent over, put his hand on my shoulder and whispered, 'You have done an outstanding job Andrew'. He was really saying, 'Well, you might now be on the pills, but if it wasn't for all the work you did earlier, we wouldn't be at this moment of glory'. I said something derogatory like, 'It's not all it's cracked up to be', enough perhaps to alert him, because ten minutes later he reappeared and asked if we could chat out in the corridor.

Outside, he asked if I had a problem with Malcolm's position. I thought I had blown my cover, so I simply said, 'There are some problems that people don't fully understand', and didn't embellish. He asked if I was going to speak, and I told him I hadn't made up my mind, that it depended on how the debate went. Back in the party room they were fifty minutes into the debate, and I knew that if I was to influence the outcome, I had to speak soon.

About five minutes later, Christopher Pyne, who was another lieutenant of Malcolm's, went outside with Michael. A few minutes after their return, Christopher casually walked up behind Malcolm and dropped a note in front of him. I have never asked what was written on that note, but I think there's a fair chance it said something like 'Andrew Robb is not enthusiastic about it'. Maybe they were suggesting Malcolm drop me down the speaking list; I don't know.

I watched, and the debate continued for another thirty minutes or so. Malcolm hadn't looked at me since he got the note. People were speaking who I knew had put up their hand after me, so I knew I had to act or I could be the second-last speaker, if not the last out of seventy-three speakers.

I ripped off a piece of paper—I didn't feel that good about doing this, but the stakes were high for our country—and wrote to Malcolm, 'The side effects of the medication I am on now make me very tired. I'd be really grateful if you could get me to my feet soon'.

He gave me a nod when he got the note. I could be totally wrong about Christopher and Michael, but I just couldn't take a risk, and I was tired—that wasn't a lie—although I had my share of adrenaline pumping and could have easily sat there for another couple of hours.

About three speakers later, Malcolm called me up and I went for it. I was given two extensions of five minutes each. You could hear a pin drop. I got a standing ovation, which doesn't happen often in the party room. I had presented facts that people could understand and I had poked holes all over their proposal.

Everyone wanted to speak, and I have never known that to happen before. Everyone knew the exact numbers in the end, as Malcolm had asked people to indicate during their comments whether they supported the negotiated agreement or not.

Malcolm can be ruthless; he just goes for broke, stares people down and walks over the top of them. He'll do anything to close a deal, and he's very effective at it. There's no doubt if I'd given him any indication of the extent of my concerns, I would have been the last speaker or he would have had people lined up to diffuse the issues. But after I spoke, there were still six hours of debate left, as it turned out. Ian and Malcolm had every opportunity to address the concerns I presented; they didn't, which said it all.

They subsequently said that my action was treacherous, but I thought it was gross treachery on their part to so misrepresent the negotiations. I still have no regrets because I felt that it was such a significant issue, and such bad and dangerous policy, being so disingenuously and cunningly rammed through our party room. There would have been many thousands of jobs lost in Australia, without any global improvement to the environment. It would have exported jobs and emissions. It was just politics.

I left the party room about half an hour after I'd spoken and was sitting in my office when Malcolm rang, during a lunch break in the debate. I got the most uncomplimentary character assessment that I've ever had. Malcolm can marshal words in a very effective way if he's looking to explain your failings as he sees them. It was water off a duck's back to me. I have known Malcolm a long time. I've got on well with him and I know what he's like. The issue was bigger than either of us. I think he had chosen me for that portfolio because I was a good bridge between the Right and the Left, and he thought the Right would listen to me but that I would do his bidding. He was wrong. I am my own man.

There was uproar after the seven and a half hours of debate, and Malcolm said he had the numbers, even though everyone knew the numbers showed a majority of thirteen against. I was back in the room by then. He told everyone, 'I am exercising my prerogative, and my judgement is that the party room supports it'. Malcolm then gave us a short, angry lecture on being part of the twenty-first century and marched off down the middle of the room. It was a dummy spit, really.

Malcolm returned at 8 p.m. after some cooler heads had spoken to him, and he was more even-tempered. He said, 'It's still my clear decision that this is the way it's going to be and there are procedures if people want to disagree with that'. In other words, you can challenge me by challenging my leadership.

The next day Kevin Andrews, to his great credit, did challenge Malcolm, and to everyone's surprise got 35 votes. They were the same 35 votes that Tony Abbott subsequently got in the first round of voting for the leadership the following Tuesday. No-one had set out to remove Malcolm as leader. The objective was to oppose the government's ETS, at least until it was clear what would and would not happen in Copenhagen. However, Malcolm chose to link his leadership irrevocably to his support for the government's ETS, irrespective of what the rest of the world was doing.

This was in total contradiction to the proposition that Malcolm had so powerfully advocated all year—that there could not be a successful national solution, only a successful global solution; that we could not go it alone. Colleagues felt they had been suckered. The only way to change the ETS policy was to change the leader. Nick Minchin led the charge.

Tony Abbott challenged Malcolm. Joe Hockey also threw his hat in the ring. After three days of bizarre twists and turns, combined with Malcolm going on television and roundly abusing some senior colleagues, particularly his Senate leader, Nick Minchin, most people entered the party room thinking that Joe Hockey would be elected. Tony won by one vote over Malcolm. Tony looked sure-footed from the moment he stepped forward to acknowledge his win.

We stopped agreeing with and apologising to the government on many issues, and started to keep the government truly accountable. Our unambiguous opposition to the government's ETS—'Say no to Rudd's great big new tax'—struck a chord with the electorate. For the first time, Kevin Rudd faced strong opposition, and he was flummoxed. In addition, Copenhagen was a disaster for Kevin and the government, leaving the world further away than ever from a global agreement on climate change.

Then, in an extraordinary ambush, Labor's faceless men orchestrated the removal of Kevin as prime minister and installed Julia Gillard. Kevin had dominated federal politics for three years, yet here he was, removed and humiliated, before even completing one term. Julia saw a brief lift in the polls before making a number of bad policy judgements of her own.

We were trending the right way in the polls when the election was called on 17 July 2010. We thought anything could happen, and it did. The last time we had a hung parliament was eighty years ago, so by any definition, it is an extraordinary position, and the fact that the so-called conservative independents gave their support to Labor made it even more so.

I was involved to some extent with the negotiations, but from the very first meeting with the crossbench independents, I felt that Tony Windsor and Rob Oakeshott were using the seventeen days to legitimise a decision that they had already made. Even at the first meeting there was a lot of *bon amie* but no discussion of substance.

We received 700 000 more votes than Labor and won more seats than Labor, yet they were in government. It was crushing; to be in Opposition is not why you go into politics. So there was deep disappointment.

On the upside, back in our electorates there was a sense among our party membership that we had come back from the train wreck nine months before, which we had. Mainly thanks to Tony Abbott, we'd come within an inch of government. They were pleased at how close we had come.

Tony has proven to be an exceptional politician. He has shown a capacity to listen, to discipline himself, to be alert to the traps that are being set and to pick his battlegrounds. Strategically, I think he's proven to be one of the most talented politicians that we've seen in the last few decades.

17

GETTING BETTER

Once Tony Abbott took over as our leader in December 2009 and was forming his Cabinet, he rang asking about my health, saying he wanted me in Shadow Cabinet.

At that stage Professor Tiller and I still hadn't found the right medication. My morning disposition continued, as did the side effects to the drugs, but as long as I had control over my work program, I could function all right. Tony and I agreed policy coordination would be a good role for me, and it didn't require any public work. It meant if there was a meeting, and I didn't feel like it, I could reschedule. It was a great opportunity, helped me feel enthusiastic and gave me something to think about over summer.

Barnaby Joyce had been appointed to Finance, and by March 2010 had started to come under excessive scrutiny for some of his comments. I've got a lot of time for Barnaby: he is an exceptionally bright fellow and he has a lot of experience. Barnaby is a leader. He has had experience working with both big and small business, and he has a good network of people. But the issue was a distraction ahead of an election. Tony decided a reshuffle was necessary and he asked if I was ready to join the Shadow ministry.

As it turned out, I had just found the magical chemical cocktail; I was feeling better in the mornings than I could ever remember. But it was still early days. Given the apparent success of the new drugs, I had privately decided that I would not seek to move back into the public arena until after the Budget, which was about six weeks away, even if I had no specific portfolio responsibilities. When Tony offered me the Finance portfolio, I gave a qualified answer and said I would get back to him quickly.

I needed time, and I needed to talk to Maureen and Professor Tiller. I hesitated because, having withdrawn from public life once, I knew that if this apparently successful pill wore off and I needed more time to sort things out, I would have to leave Shadow Cabinet again, which would be the end of my political career. I couldn't keep coming and going, because people would lose confidence that I had overcome my illness. My only concern was that I was taking the risk of returning too early.

Professor Tiller made an astute observation. He said, 'There's an election coming up; you've had five weeks of feeling well; there's every prospect you could continue that way. If you don't re-establish yourself before the election, you won't be able to participate strongly during the election. If you don't take this political opportunity, it mightn't come again for a while, or ever, whether you are well or not'. I was keen, and Maureen and Professor Tiller encouraged me, so I rang Tony and said, 'I'm on', and I've gone from strength to strength.

I had no sense of what was going to happen when I originally went public with my condition. I had hoped for a sympathetic response, but I hadn't expected the hundreds of emails that started to pour in. Overwhelmingly they were positive, but there were a few telling me I was a weak character and should get out of politics. That had been my own misconception for years: that depression was seen as a personality defect, and anyone known to be suffering from it would not be trusted. But overwhelmingly most people were supportive, or asked for my assistance. I was also struck by the number of people, a dozen or so, who are captains of industry—well-known figures in the community, some of them running organisations with tens of thousands of employees—who sent me messages, either a text message or a short note or email, saying something to the effect of: 'Welcome to the club'.

Kevin Rudd rang me the morning the Laurie Oakes article was published. He was on an aircraft to Washington. I appreciated the contact. Penny Wong rang later that morning from Washington and was very considerate. All my colleagues were sympathetic, positive and concerned. Through social media I can cop some unkind comments if people don't like what I am saying; they will tweet that I must have forgotten to take my pills or that the medication must be making me hypo. Cheap shots.

It is nearly twenty-four months since I went public, and still people refer to it one way or another wherever I am. They will cry out in the middle of a function of 400 people, just wanting to talk about their own battle with depression or how it has affected someone close to them.

I had been uncertain what the reaction would be to my announce-ment, but it has been a wonderful experience. I thought it might help people, but I didn't know whether people would be sympathetic or if it would mark me for life. But in the last eighteen months I have had more parliamentary responsibility than I've ever had, and for the first time I am enjoying it. I don't feel people are holding my condition against me. Most people realise I have an illness, respect the fact I have it under control and accept that now I am well.

In finally dealing with my own depression I hoped to demonstrate that, in many cases, if you confront it, persist until you find good professional advice that suits you and then show patience in finding the answer to your problem, the results can exceed your expectations. Usually you can stay in your job, taking on, if you wish, even more responsibility than you previously carried, and in most instances doing all this without telling the world. Tackling and managing your depressive condition can give even greater meaning to your life.

My maiden speech to federal parliament on 29 November 2004 started with the following observation:

> From as early as I can remember, my mother and father instilled in me and my eight brothers and sisters that opportunity and freedom would come through education, personal responsibility and self-belief: that our destiny was largely in our own hands—how hard we studied and worked, the opportunities we took, how we dealt with people.
>
> I grew to believe that I was responsible for charting my own course—that I was free to follow my dreams, make my own mistakes, take the consequences of my decisions.
>
> Importantly, my parents never seemed to convey any resentment or jealousy that others might have more than we had; there was no chip on the shoulder, rather a notion of 'blue sky', a sense that if we really wanted what others had—whatever that might be—then the opportunity was there in Australia to achieve it. Ambition was presented as a good thing, something to be nurtured and supported, and not only in sport.
>
> I embraced these simple truths as a philosophy, elements that I later came to see as best captured by the Liberal Party philosophy.

I believe that my life has been conditioned and driven by these principles. I have taken responsibility for dealing with my lot in the morning, sustained by a strong sense of self-belief and an urge to grab the promised opportunities and freedoms.

I have not been disappointed. I have had a great life to date, blessed with interesting and challenging work, and I have a wonderful wife, three great children, two loving parents and eight siblings who are real friends.

Now that I finally have the courage to tackle my demons, to confront the perceived stigma of depression, it can only get better. In my case, I suspect that without dealing with the inner suffering in the morning, some of the personal growth I've achieved and resilience I've developed may not have been possible.

I believe that we are all born with our own unique sets of talents and personal circumstances, and that we each have a responsibility to achieve what we should, within the limits of those talents and environment. Striving and struggling to reach our own potential is what gives meaning to our lives. And it is what dictates the uniqueness and dignity of each person.

The conclusion to my maiden speech remains my strong view:

> True happiness, true freedom, comes from achievement;
> using whatever God-given talents we have to chart our own
> course, to take the consequences of our decisions, to have
> a go. If we do this, success and happiness will follow.

Politics teaches you that life is meaningful; you see so many people who have found meaning in their lives, people who have realised that life is still expecting something from them despite their circumstances.

My achievement in finding a solution to my morning affliction has given me greater freedom and opportunity. For the foreseeable future, the opportunity I was striving for has closed.

GETTING BETTER

But it still remains that when you are sounded out to stand for leader of your political party, there can only be one answer. And I would now have no hesitation to give it.

WHERE TO FIND HELP FOR
MOOD DISORDERS

There are many support options, telephone helplines and websites where you can find out more information or get help. Some are listed below.

Someone to talk to

You could speak to your local doctor, psychologist, psychiatrist or community health care worker. Also consider counsellors, close friends, family members or family friends, a neighbour, police officers, religious or community leaders.

Phone support:

Lifeline Australia	13 11 14
Mental Health Information Service	1300 794 991
SANE Australia	1800 187 263
Rural Mental Health Support Line	1800 201 123
MensLine	1300 789 978
Kids Helpline	1800 551 800

The Black Dog Institute has a range of helpful fact sheets on their web site including 'What to expect from a mental health consultation' and 'Helping someone who has a mood disorder—for family and friends'. See blackdoginstitute.org.au/factsheets

Specialist services

beyondblue

beyondblue is a national, independent, not-for-profit organisation with a key goal of raising community awareness about depression and anxiety, and reducing stigmas associated with the illness.
beyondblue.org.au

Black Dog Institute

The Black Dog Institute is a not-for-profit organisation offering specialist expertise in depression and bipolar disorder. Activities include research, clinics (on referral), eHealth initiatives, support groups, professional education and community awareness.
blackdoginstitute.org.au

Useful websites

arafmi.org
ARAFMI (Association of Relatives And Friends of the Mentally Ill) provides a range of services to families, carers and friends of people with a mental illness across NSW.

beyondblue.org.au
The national depression initiative.

biteback.org.au
A youth website created by the Black Dog Institute.

blackdoginstitute.org.au
Specialist expertise in depression and bipolar disorder.

carersnsw.asn.au
Provides carer support kits, telephone assistance, support groups and other resources.

depressionet.org.au
Created by Australians who have had personal experiences with depression.

goodtherapy.com.au
This website includes a directory of practitioners and a calendar of upcoming events and workshops.

inspire.org.au
The Inspire Foundation exists to help young people lead happier lives.

lifeline.org.au
Information and where to find services in your area.

mentalhealth.asn.au
Provides information, support and education to people who are affected by mental illness, or who seek to improve their emotional wellbeing.

moodgym.com.au
Learn cognitive behaviour therapy skills to prevent and cope with depression.

reachout.com
A web-based service that aims to improve the mental health and wellbeing of young people aged 14–25 years.

sane.org
Online fact sheets and information.

ACKNOWLEDGEMENTS

It has turned out to be a very positive experience for me to reflect on my challenges with Churchill's 'Black Dog'. In my case it was a little black dog for several decades, but one that grew larger as I got older.

I sincerely hope that my experiences, where I was in denial for forty-three of the last forty-five years, may encourage others to confront a depressive condition they know or suspect they are enduring.

The inspiration, belief and opportunity to achieve these outcomes was provided by the ever effervescent Louise Adler, CEO and Publisher-in-Chief of Melbourne University Publishing. I am extremely grateful to Louise. I suggest that no aspiring author should knock back her long lunches at The European—and beware a teetotaller's encouragement!

To Maureen, my elegant and wonderful wife of thirty-five years, I am extremely indebted. She has kept my feet on the ground while providing wise advice, support and encouragement when required.

Our three children, Tom, Joe and Pip, and now their partners, Jill, Claire and Andrew, have given great joy and meaning to our lives. My quietness in the mornings doesn't appear to have set them back.

Vanessa Konig, my PA, and Cameron Hill, my Chief-of-Staff, have provided invaluable professional and moral support. They have

ACKNOWLEDGEMENTS

helped me juggle and carry out the heavy workload of my day (and night) job while I penned the book, often in the early hours. I toyed with calling it *Midnight Special* because so much of it was written after that hour.

The book owes much to the advice and efforts of MUP's Associate Publisher, Sally Heath. Her patience, persistence and expertise hopefully are rewarded with a worthwhile publication. Many thanks.

Diane Leyman, Senior Editor and Helen Koehne, as editor, also made a highly professional and valuable contribution.

I will be forever grateful to Professor John Tiller, Jeff Kennett and Dr David Cunnington for helping me successfully confront my demons and get on with my life.

Finally, my gratitude to Professor Gordon Parker, the esteemed Executive Director of the Black Dog Institute in Sydney, for allowing me to reproduce his file of organisations that can help those seeking to deal with some form of mental health problem. It is an invaluable reference.

INDEX

INDEX

INDEX